Computers and Medicine

Bruce I. Blum, *Editor*

Computers and Medicine

Perry L. Miller
Editor

Selected Topics in Medical Artificial Intelligence

With 37 Illustrations

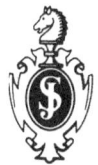

Springer-Verlag
New York Berlin Heidelberg
London Paris Tokyo

Perry L. Miller, M.D., Ph.D.
Department of Anesthesiology
Yale University School of Medicine
New Haven, Connecticut 06510
USA

Series Editor
Bruce I. Blum
Applied Physics Laboratory
The Johns Hopkins University
Laurel, Maryland 20707
USA

LIBRARY OF CONGRESS
Library of Congress Cataloging-in-Publication Data

Selected topics in medical artificial intelligence / edited by Perry
  L. Miller.
      p.   cm.—(Computers and medicine)
    Includes bibliographies and index.
    ISBN-13:978-1-4613-8779-4
    1. Artificial intelligence—Medical applications.   2. Medicine—
Data processing.   I. Miller, Perry L.   II. Series: Computers and
medicine (New York, N.Y.)
  R859.7.A78S44   1988
  610'.28'563—dc19   88-16338
                                                          CIP

© 1988 by Springer-Verlag New York Inc.
Softcover reprint of the hardcover 1st edition 1988

Typeset by David E. Seham Associates, Metuchen, New Jersey.

9 8 7 6 5 4 3 2 1

ISBN-13:978-1-4613-8779-4   e-ISBN-13:978-1-4613-8777-0
DOI: 10.1007/978-1-4613-8777-0

Series Preface

Computer technology has impacted the practice of medicine in dramatic ways. Imaging techniques provide noninvasive tools which alter the diagnostic process. Sophisticated monitoring equipment presents new levels of detail for both patient management and research. In most of these technology applications, the computer is embedded in the device; its presence is transparent to the user.

There is also a growing number of applications in which the health care provider directly interacts with a computer. In many cases, these applications are limited to administrative functions, e.g., office practice management, location of hospital patients, appointments, and scheduling. Nevertheless, there also are instances of patient care functions such as results reporting, decision support, surveillance, and reminders.

This series, Computers and Medicine, will focus upon the direct use of information systems as it relates to the medical community. After twenty-five years of experimentation and experience, there are many tested applications which can be implemented economically using the current generation of computers. Moreover, the falling cost of computers suggests that there will be even more extensive use in the near future. Yet there is a gap between current practice and the state-of-the-art.

This lag in the diffusion of technology results from a combination of two factors. First, there are few sources designed to assist practitioners in learning what the new technology can do. Secondly, because the potential is not widely understood, there is a limited marketplace for some of the more advanced applications; this, in turn, limits commercial interest in the development of new products.

In the next decade, one can expect the field of medical information science to establish a better understanding of the role of computers in medicine. Furthermore, those entering the health care professions already will have had some formal training in computer science. For the near term, however, there is a clear need for books designed to illustrate how

computers can assist in the practice of medicine. For without these col-
lections, it will be very difficult for the practitioner to learn about a technology which certainly will alter his or her approach to medicine.

And that is the purpose of this series: the presentation of readings about
the interaction of computers and medicine. The primary objectives are to
describe the current state-of-the-art and to orient medical and health
professionals and students with little or no experience with computer applications. We hope that this series will help in the rational transfer of
computer technology to medical care.

Laurel, Maryland   BRUCE BLUM

Contents

II. Knowledge Acquisition and Verification

III. Evaluation

Contributors

Robert L. Blum, M.D., Ph.D.
Research Associate, Department of Computer Science, Stanford University, Stanford, California, USA

Steven J. Blumenfrucht
Medical Student, Yale University School of Medicine, New Haven, Connecticut, USA

David M. Combs
Scientific Programmer, Medical Computer Science Group, Stanford University School of Medicine, Stanford, California, USA

Gregory F. Cooper, M.D., Ph.D.
Research Associate, Medical Computer Science Group, Stanford University School of Medicine, Stanford, California, USA

Modestino G. Criscitiello, M.D.
Professor of Medicine, Department of Medicine, Tufts University School of Medicine, Boston, Massachusetts, USA

Lawrence M. Fagan, M.D., Ph.D.
Senior Research Associate, Department of Medicine, Stanford University School of Medicine, Stanford, California, USA

Paul R. Fisher, M.D.
Assistant Professor, Department of Diagnostic Radiology, Yale University School of Medicine, New Haven, Connecticut, USA

Allen Ginsberg, Ph.D.
Member of Technical Staff, Knowledge Systems Research Department, AT&T Bell Laboratories, Holmdel, New Jersey, USA

Robert L. Jayes
  Research Fellow, Division of Clinical Decision Making, Department
  of Medicine, New England Medical Center and Tufts University
  School of Medicine, Boston, Massachusetts, USA

Lawrence C. Kingsland III, Ph.D.
  Chief, Computer Science Branch, Lister Hill National Center for
  Biomedical Communications, National Library of Medicine.
  Bethesda, Maryland, USA

Yong Bok Lee, Ph.D.
  Special Advisor to the President, Korean Electric Power
  Corporation, Seoul, Korea

William J. Long, Ph.D.
  Principal Research Associate, Laboratory for Computer Science,
  Massachusetts Institute of Technology, Cambridge, Massachusetts,
  USA

Nicolaas J.I. Mars, Ph.D.
  Professor of Computer Science, University of Twente, Enschede,
  The Netherlands

Perry L. Miller, M.D., Ph.D.
  Associate Professor of Anesthesiology, Yale University School of
  Medicine, New Haven, Connecticut, USA

Randolph A. Miller, M.D.
  Associate Professor of Medicine, University of Pittsburgh School of
  Medicine, Pittsburgh, Pennsylvania, USA

Mark A. Musen, M.D.
  Assistant Professor of Medicine, Stanford University School of
  Medicine, Stanford, California, USA

Shapur Naimi, Ph.D.
  Associate Professor of Medicine, Tufts University School of
  Medicine, Boston, Massachusetts, USA

Yoh-Han Pao, Ph.D.
  Professor of Electrical Engineering and Computer Science, Case
  Western Reserve University, Cleveland, Ohio, USA

Ronnie C. Parker, M.D.
  Assistant Professor of Medicine, University of Pittsburgh School of
  Medicine, Pittsburgh, Pennsylvania, USA

Ramesh S. Patil, Ph.D.
Assistant Professor of Computer Science, Massachusetts Institute of
Technology, Cambridge, Massachusetts, USA

Peter Politakis, Ph.D.
Manager, Software Engineering, Digital Equipment Corporation,
Hudson, Massachusetts, USA

James A. Reggia, M.D., Ph.D.
Associate Professor, Departments of Neurology and Computer
Science, University of Maryland, Baltimore, Maryland USA

Glenn D. Rennels
Resident in Anesthesiology, Stanford University School of Medicine,
Stanford, California, USA

John R. Rose
Graduate Student, Department of Computer Science, SUNY at
Stony Brook, New York, USA

Michael Rothschild
Medical Student, Yale University School of Medicine, New Haven,
Connecticut, USA

Oksana Senyk, M.D., Ph.D.
Assistant Professor of Medicine, Tufts University School of
Medicine, Boston, Massachusetts, USA

Edward H. Shortliffe, M.D., Ph.D.
Associate Professor of Medicine, Stanford University School of
Medicine, Stanford, California, USA

Stephen W. Smoliar, Ph.D.
Senior Research Scientist, University of Southern California
Information Sciences Institute, Marina del Rey, California, USA

Frank E. Stockdale, M.D., Ph.D.
Professor of Medicine, Stanford University School of Medicine,
Stanford, California, USA

William R. Swartout, Ph.D.
Senior Research Scientist, University of Southern California
Information Sciences Institute, Marina del Rey, California, USA

Henry A. Swett, M.D.
  Associate Professor, Department of Diagnostic Radiology, Yale
  University School of Medicine, New Haven, Connecticut, USA

Joan D. Walton
  Research Assistant, Medical Computer Science Group, Stanford
  University School of Medicine, Stanford, California, USA

Sholom M. Weiss, Ph.D.
  Research Professor, Rutgers University, Department of Computer
  Science, New Brunswick, New Jersey, USA

Gregory Weltin, M.D.
  Assistant Professor, Department of Diagnostic Radiology, Yale
  University School of Medicine, New Haven, Connecticut, USA

Lawrence E. Widman, M.D., Ph.D.
  Assistant Professor of Medicine, University of Texas Health Science
  Center at San Antonio, Texas, USA

1
Artificial Intelligence in Medicine: An Emerging Discipline

Perry L. Miller

Over the past 25 years there have been a wide variety of computer applications in medicine. They include financial and accounting systems, clinical data management systems, biomedical engineering applications, clinical decision support systems, and many more. This book addresses a particular type of medical computer research, the application of artificial intelligence (AI) techniques in medicine.

Artificial intelligence is a subfield of computer science that can be loosely defined as the science of developing computer systems that exhibit "intelligent" behavior. In medicine, AI systems have typically been designed to assist in patient care, i.e., to help diagnose and treat disease. It rapidly became clear that such systems require a great deal of medical knowledge in order to perform these tasks effectively and that much of this knowledge must be extracted from experts in the field. As a result, these AI-based computer systems have come to be called "knowledge-based systems" or "expert systems." The field itself is often referred to as artificial intelligence in medicine (AIM).

The task of giving effective advice to the physician has turned out to be challenging for reasons discussed later in this chapter. As a result, most AIM projects are currently still in the basic research and prototype stages. A small number of AIM systems are just starting to move into the practical clinical arena.

Artificial Intelligence in Medicine

The field of AIM has evolved over the past 15 years as an active and growing discipline. The field was born during the late 1960s and early 1970s with the implementation of a number of AI-based systems at several academic centers. These systems include: MYCIN[1] at Stanford, which deals with infectious disease; CASNET[2] at Rutgers, whose domain is ophthalmology; INTERNIST[3] at Pittsburgh, which embraces the whole of internal medicine; and PIP[4] at MIT, which handles renal disease. These initial projects have spawned follow-on projects, and AIM research has spread to other institutions. The work performed during the first decade of this research has been surveyed in several articles and books.[5–8]

During the years since the early systems were implemented, a number of interesting developments have occurred. One development has been that the field of AI itself has grown explosively and has been transformed from an academic curiosity to a field with robust industrial and commercial activity. It is interesting that a great deal of the impetus behind the commercial growth of AI as a whole arose initially from the early research performed in domains of medicine.

Another development is that the field of medical AI has matured. This maturity is reflected by the fact that a range of specific topics for AIM research have emerged, including such research topics as:

Causal modeling
Strategic reasoning
Explanation
Knowledge acquisition and verification
Validation and evaluation of AIM systems
Anatomic reasoning
Temporal reasoning
Reasoning from multiple sources of knowledge
Intelligent computer-assisted instruction (ICAI)
Integration of natural language processing with medical expert systems
Integration of Medical Decision Analysis (MDA) and AI techniques

Certain of these topics are closely tied to unique characteristics of medicine, e.g., the evaluation of AIM systems and the merging of MDA and AI techniques. Many of these topics, however, apply not only to medical AI but to AI research in general.

This book contains groups of chapters that address several of these research topics. Most of the chapters are based on papers that were originally presented at invited sessions of the annual Symposium on Computer Applications in Medical Care (SCAMC). The SCAMC conference is held each fall, usually in Washington, DC, and currently attracts approximately 2500 attendees. As a former member of the SCAMC Program Committee, the editor organized several invited sessions on topics thought to be of particular interest. The invited sessions typically included an overview paper summarizing the topic as a whole, followed by several papers describing specific research projects.

Nature of Computer Science Research: Using the Computer as a Laboratory to Explore Ideas

The projects described in this book are examples of computer science research. This type of research may be unfamiliar to many readers. It is certainly different from much of the experimental research (in either the laboratory or the clinic) familiar to many in medicine.

Computer science research frequently involves *exploratory programming:* using the computer as a "laboratory" to explore complex system design issues. The goal of this research is *not* to implement polished, operational systems but, rather, to take a set of ideas and intuitions that may initially be unstructured and use the computer to help make those ideas more concrete. Thus the computer provides:

1. A mechanism to obtain feedback concerning one's thinking
2. A vehicle to stimulate further thinking
3. A crucible to test the validity, consistency, and completeness of one's ideas incrementally as they evolve

Computer science research is successful to the extent, for example, that it:

1. Raises important new issues and questions
2. Demonstrates new potential solutions to interesting problems
3. Demonstrates the limitations of particular approaches and solutions

Computer science research therefore involves the iterative refinement of ideas. In a sense, one might compare performing computer science research to climbing a mountain. The project is an arduous process in and of itself, and a number of interesting problems may need to be solved just to carry it out successfully. At the same time, however, the most rewarding aspect of the whole project may be the view from the top of the mountain when the climb is completed. Once one has finished a computer science research project, there are typically a number of interesting further questions that could be addressed. There is also a much better appreciation of the advantages and limitations of the approach taken. In addition, the researcher frequently develops insights about completely different, possibly more powerful solutions to the various problems encountered.

As a result, when reporting computer science research, it is important not only to describe what has been done but also to discuss some of the interesting "lessons learned." In other words, one should not only describe the path taken up the mountain and why one chose that path, the view from the top should also be described.

What Is AIM Research?

The field of AIM spans a considerable range, from basic research to applied projects. This section outlines three general types of AIM project.

Basic AI Research

At one end of the AIM spectrum is basic AI research performed in a medical domain. Basic AI research addresses fundamental issues in developing "intelligent" computer-based capabilities. Among the issues addressed by basic AI research are the following.

Knowledge representation: how best to represent complex real-world knowledge so it can be used in sophisticated ways

Learning: how to design a computer system so it can update and modify its own knowledge, either from observation or experience, or because it is explicitly told new information

Planning: the various issues involved in efficiently identifying and evaluating alternative approaches to a problem

Temporal reasoning: being able to model a system as it changes over time, so a computer can reason intelligently about that system

Spatial reasoning: modeling spatial relations in a flexible way so that a computer can reason about them in a general fashion

Natural language understanding: dealing with the complex problems of understanding a human language, e.g., English

Basic AI research of this sort, of course, can be carried into a diverse range of domains beyond medicine. Nevertheless, the inherent complexity of medicine and of medical information processing makes medicine a rich domain for exploring basic AI research issues.

Applications of AI Techniques

At the other end of the AIM spectrum is the straightforward application of AI techniques in medicine. An example of such a project is using an existing rule interpreter to create a rule-based system for a diagnostic task, where no new computer system design issues are explored.

As the field of AIM matures and the various techniques developed become well established, one can anticipate that more and more projects will be undertaken that are not research projects, at least not from a computer science perspective. A word of caution, however, may be appropriate. Domains of medicine are notoriously idiosyncratic and may be different from one another in their computational implications. As a result, a project that starts out as the "mere" application of AI techniques in medicine may well evolve into a more ambitious research project as unexpected features of the domain are encountered.

Research in Medical Expert Systems

Medical expert system research sits at the intersection between basic AI research and the application of AI techniques. One is tempted to make an analogy between "pure science" and engineering. Indeed, expert system research has been called "knowledge engineering." An equally cogent argument can be made, however, that expert system research is one sub-area of basic AI research.

However one characterizes the field of expert system research, it is clear that it is a robust research area with many complex questions remaining to be answered. The field addresses many issues, including: (1) how best to represent real-world knowledge in the machine; (2) how to manipulate that knowledge for such purposes as explanation, knowledge acquisition, verification, and updating; and (3) how best to evaluate medical expert systems. This book centers around research issues such as these.

Challenges Medical AI Faces Today

A wide variety of expert systems have been developed in diverse areas of medicine. Indeed, as mentioned previously, much of the current explosive industrial and commercial activity in the implementation of expert systems has evolved to a large degree from basic research performed in domains of medicine. Despite all this research activity, few AI-based medical systems have yet achieved practical, operational status.

At the same time, expert system technology has been widely and successfully applied in many domains outside of medicine. This situation raises an interesting question. Why should medicine be such a productive area for the development of expert system technology that has been applied in many other domains, yet that has still to be widely applied within medicine itself?

The answer to this question is simple: Medicine is a complex domain. This complexity forces researchers to develop powerful, general, flexible tools to attack medical problems. Once these tools are developed, however, they are much more easily applied to simpler, more structured problems. The complexity of medicine stems from many factors, including the

1. Complexity of the human body and of human disease processes
2. Relatively shallow level of knowledge we currently have concerning most diseases
3. Huge amount of knowledge relevant to even a constrained subspecialty area of medicine
4. Lack of familiarity with computers on the part of many health care personnel
5. Pressured time demands on the practicing physician
6. Legal implications of giving advice regarding patient care

Diverse Nature of Medical Knowledge

The diverse nature of medical knowledge is best illustrated by comparing medical decision-making to decision-making in a more structured domain. For example, one might compare the diagnosis of human illness with the diagnosis of faults in an automobile. The biggest difference between these two domains arises because an automobile is a *manufactured* device. The various pieces are specifically designed for particular functions, and most if not all faults can be understood in terms of these known functions.

In contrast, the underlying problems in medicine are much less well understood. Although the mechanisms of some disease processes are reasonably clear, such situations are relatively rare. Even when underlying mechanisms of disease are suspected, there are usually several competing hypotheses, none of which may be correct. In the face of all this partial and incomplete information, the practicing physician is forced to utilize a broad spectrum of different types of knowledge for guidance in patient care.

Superficial relations. Much medical knowledge is represented as fairly superficial relations that have been compiled over years of clinical practice by many physicians. For diagnosis, for example, sets of clinical signs and symptoms are linked to the various diseases in which they tend to occur. For treatment, established approaches have evolved to structure the management of particular medical problems. Although there is a great deal of rote memorization required to master this material, there is also much judgment and skill needed to apply the knowledge intelligently to a particular patient's care.

Causal knowledge. As discussed previously, there are a limited number of medical domains where fairly detailed causal mechanisms are understood. There are also many other domains where causal hypotheses (often conflicting) exist. Such knowledge clearly plays a role in medical reasoning.

Case-based knowledge. A great deal of the knowledge physicians use in patient care is structured around previous cases they have seen or have heard described.

Clinical literature. Numerous studies are published that evaluate the relative efficacy of different approaches to a particular medical problem. Medical practice may shift dramatically based on such studies. In this regard, it is necessary for the clinician not only to know the general results of a study but also to have a critical understanding of the study's strengths, weaknesses, and clinical implications, as well as its relation to previous studies.

As a result, medical practice rests on a wide range of different types of knowledge, and the physician must be able to integrate these areas when undertaking a patient's care. To offer clinically robust advice, an expert system is ideally able to integrate this diversity of knowledge as well.

Latitude for Variation and Subjective Judgment in Medical Practice

Another challenging facet of medical practice is the tremendous latitude for practice variation and for subjective judgment to influence patient care.

Practice variation. There are frequently several ways to approach a problem in medicine. Although certain approaches are usually clearly wrong, it is seldom the case that a single approach is clearly "right." The widespread variation in medical practice stems from a variety of factors. Different training institutions frequently advocate different styles of practice and different approaches. Patterns of care differ in different geographic areas and at different hospitals within a single area. Moreover, medicine is constantly in flux. New techniques are developed and are incorporated into practice at different rates. Some become an established part of medicine, whereas others pass eventually into obscurity.

Subjective judgment. There is also widespread latitude for subjective judgment in medical decision-making. A physician must frequently assess the severity and urgency of a patient's problems and base the treatment on these judgments. Such assessments are often subjective in nature, and different physicians may well be led to different decisions regarding the same patient's care. Neither a computer nor another physician can necessarily tell a physician what to do.

In the face of this widespread latitude for practice variation and subjective judgment, a traditional expert system that in effect tries to tell a physician what to do may have little value. To help deal with this problem, several projects have explored a different approach to bringing computer-based advice to the physician—a *critiquing* approach.[9] A critiquing system first asks the physician to describe the patient and to outline how he or she contemplates approaching the patient's management. The critiquing system then discusses that plan, thereby structuring its advice around the physician's own thinking and style of practice.

Lack of an Objective "Gold Standard"

A related problem in the design of medical expert systems is particularly evident when one undertakes to validate a system's knowledge base to ensure its accuracy, completeness, and consistency. The problem is that for most domains of medicine there is no "gold standard" that defines optimal care.

This problem arises not only because of issues of practice variation and subjective judgment, as discussed above, but also because experts in the field may frankly disagree as to the best approach to certain problems. As a result, it can be difficult to define an appropriate standard against which to measure a system's performance. Chapter 15 discusses this problem in more detail.

Pressured Nature of Medical Practice

Another challenge is the pressured nature of medical practice, where a patient's medical problems are typically dealt with in a fast, expeditious fashion. Working in this environment, the physician rarely tolerates a computer system that makes major demands on his time. In this way the inherent nature of medical practice itself presents a major obstacle to the widespread use of medical expert systems.

Physician Acceptance of Computers

A related problem is that of acceptance of computer technology by physicians. Most physicians are not familiar with computers and may not be comfortable using them. Becoming comfortable with computer technology requires a significant commitment of time and energy. Unfortunately, the practicing physician is already inundated by a constant stream of new medical knowledge. These demands cut into time that might otherwise be used to learn about computers.

Looking to the Future

The previous section outlined some of the challenges the field of AIM faces. None of these difficulties is insurmountable. They do imply, however, that the sophisticated integration of computer technology in support of decision-making in medicine will take longer than in many other areas of life. Fortunately, a number of factors can help overcome these difficulties.

1. *Increasing computer sophistication of physicians.* Even though the typical medical practitioner may not be familiar with computer technology, many medical students being trained today are indeed comfortable with it. Also, medical computing topics are increasingly being included in medical school curricula. In addition, in the near future it is planned that parts of the medical National Board examination will be administered interactively using computers. As a result, the problem of physician acceptance of computer technology will become less and less of a problem as time passes.

2. *Increasing number of researchers fully trained in both computer science and medicine.* In the early phases of AIM research, communication between the two cultures—computer science and clinical medicine—represented a major impediment to successful research. Computer specialists often had difficulty fully appreciating the clinical environment, and clinicians often had trouble appreciating the strengths and limitations of computers. More recently, there are increasing numbers of researchers

fully trained in both fields. Such individuals tend to have a unique advantage in being able to identify problems that are interesting from both a computer and a clinical point of view and in helping keep a research project focused productively.

3. *Computerization of clinical data.* Computers are increasingly being used to store clinical data, in both ambulatory information systems and hospital information systems. As more and more clinical data are stored on the computer, it will greatly facilitate the use of expert systems. First, the physician-user may already be interacting with the computer, e.g., inspecting laboratory values or entering orders. Second, if much of the clinical information the expert system needs is already online, that system's interaction with the physician may be greatly streamlined.

4. *Advances in computer hardware.* Another factor is the rapid pace at which computer hardware continues to develop, coupled with dramatic decreases in cost. The type of hardware needed to accomplish the sophisticated processing required by many expert systems is becoming increasingly affordable. Moreover, the development of inexpensive yet powerful graphics interfaces make it easier for the physician to interact comfortably and efficiently with the machine.

Of course, none of these changes will lead to the widespread use of medical expert systems without a major effort invested in further AIM research. It is encouraging, however, to look to the future knowing that the whole environment in which AIM systems will be used is undergoing a transformation and that medical practice will be increasingly able to accommodate the power and potential AIM research will ultimately be able to offer.

References

1. Shortliffe EH: Computer-Based Medical Consultations: MYCIN. New York: Elsevier, 1976.
2. Kulikowski C, Weiss SM: Representation of expert knowledge for consultation: the CASNET and EXPERT projects. In Szolovits P (ed): Artificial Intelligence in Medicine. Boulder, CO: Westview Press, 1982.
3. Miller RA, Pople HE, Meyers JD: Internist-I, an experimental computer-based diagnostic consultant for general internal medicine. N Engl J Med 307:468, 1982.
4. Pauker SG, Gorry GA, Kassirer JP, Schwartz WB: Towards the simulation of clinical cognition: taking a present illness by computer. Am J Med 60:981, 1976.
5. Kulikowski C: Artificial intelligence methods and systems for medical consultation. IEEE Trans PAMI PAMI-2:464, 1980.
6. Shortliffe EH, Buchannan BG, Feigenbaum EA: Knowledge engineering for medical decision making: a review of computer-based clinical decision aids. Proc IEEE 67:1207, 1979.

7. Clancey WJ, Shortliffe EH (eds): Readings in Medical Artificial Intelligence: The First Decade. Reading, MA: Addison-Wesley, 1984.
8. Szolovits P (ed): Artificial Intelligence in Medicine. Boulder, CO: Westview Press, 1982.
9. Miller PL: Expert Critiquing Systems: Practice-Based Medical Consultation by Computer. New York: Springer Verlag, 1986.

2
Causal Models for Medical Artificial Intelligence

Perry L. Miller and Paul R. Fisher

Introduction

A large number of expert systems have been developed using artificial intelligence (AI) techniques to assist in medical diagnosis and treatment.[1,2] Most of these systems involve "surface models" of their domains rather than "causal models" of the underlying physiologic and pathophysiologic processes. Such a surface model links sets of patient findings with different diseases to assist diagnosis or defines the clinical conditions for which particular treatments are recommended.

Several projects have explored how more fundamental knowledge of the domain might help a computer reason about medical problems. Much of this work has focused on causal models: exploring how such models might best be implemented and how they might best be integrated into medical expert systems. This work raises a number of interesting questions, including:

1. How well suited is the domain of medicine for causal modeling?
2. To what extent do physicians use causal models when performing patient care?
3. To what extent do physicians use causal models when explaining and justifying their clinical decisions?
4. How might a causal model be used by a computer to help a physician perform patient care?
5. What other types of fundamental knowledge might be useful in medical expert systems?

An underlying motivation for developing causal models is the conviction that such a model may let the computer understand its domain more profoundly and therefore reason about the domain in a more general fashion. One problem with applying causal models in medicine is that for many diseases the underlying causal mechanisms are either unknown or controversial.

From *Proceedings, 11th Symposium on Computer Applications in Medical Care*, pp. 17–22, © 1987, Institute of Electrical and Electronics Engineers, Inc. Reprinted with permission.

Research Issues Underlying Medical Causal Modeling

Qualitative Causal Models

Any computer program that represents the causal relations between the components of a mechanical or biologic system is in some sense a causal model. Many computer simulation programs fall within this general definition. They are usually mathematical models used to help one better understand a system's general behavior or to predict the system's behavior under specific conditions. Although mathematical simulation programs frequently incorporate causal relations, these relations are usually buried in the program itself and are not used by the computer to reason explicitly about the behavior of the model.

In contrast, in the AI systems described herein, the various causal relations are *explicit* in the sense that the computer can inspect them, manipulate them, and explore their implications. Another characteristic of AI causal models is that many are *qualitative* causal models. In a qualitative model, variables are given qualitative values. For example, in a model of the cardiovascular system, variables such as cardiac output, blood pressure, heart rate, and systemic vascular resistance would have non-numeric values, e.g., "normal," "slightly elevated," "high," and "very high." Such a qualitative model differs from the conventional (quantitative) simulation programs mentioned above where all variables have numeric values.

The motivation for developing qualitative models stems in part from a belief that they may more accurately mirror human reasoning. Also, by expressing variables in symbolic terms, qualitative models may make it easier for systems to reason explicitly about the implications of the various causal relations involved.

Dealing with Interacting Forces in Qualitative Modeling

The use of a qualitative model forces the system designer to confront a number of difficulties that do not occur when building quantitative simulation models. A major problem is how to deal with situations where forces conflict or otherwise interact.

For example, in a model of the cardiovascular system there are several causal forces that may make a patient's blood pressure (BP) increase, and several forces that may make it decrease. In a *quantitative* model, when several such forces act simultaneously the various mathematical equations define exactly what will happen to the BP: whether it will remain constant, rise, or fall, and to exactly what degree.

In a *qualitative* model, however, it is unclear how best to resolve the effects of interacting forces. With a simple qualitative model, when several conflicting forces act on a variable, all the system can say is, for example,

"BP may rise, fall, or remain unchanged." Such a simple qualitative model would therefore be of little use for the cardiovascular system, where not only are there multiple conflicting forces but the function of the whole system relies on multiple homeostatic feedback loops.

Because such feedback loops exist throughout medicine, a medical causal model must be prepared to deal with this problem. As a result, the problem of how best to handle interacting forces remains a central research issue for medical qualitative modeling.

Temporal Aspects of Causality

A further component of causality involves time. Time is an integral part of causal relations. A causal process takes place over a period of time that may be discrete or continuous. If it is discrete, its duration may be variable. Also, there may well be *delays* between the event that initiates a causal change and the subsequent event that is "caused." Depending on the domain, on the type of causal relations in the domain, and on the type of reasoning the system is to perform, a causal model may need to be built on an underlying model of time and temporal relations.

Characterizing the Nature of Causality

Different causal relations may have a range of characteristics. Certain of these characteristics have already been mentioned, e.g., that the effects of some causes are discrete events in time whereas others are continuous, that some causes involve significant delays while others do not.

Other distinctions include the following: (1) Some causal relations are direct (if event A occurs, event B will definitely occur), whereas others are potentiating (if event A occurs, event B may occur). (2) Event A may need to be present while event B occurs, or event A may need only to be present to initiate event B. Depending on the particular model and domain, it may be necessary to categorize the nature of causality in various ways to allow the computer to reason about causal relations intelligently.

Modeling Causal Relations at Different Levels of Detail

Another interesting aspect of causality is that it can be modeled at different levels of detail. This situation can be seen clearly when a child keeps asking "Why?" For example, "Why did the car stop?" "Because I stepped on the brakes." "Why did that make the car stop?" etc. Such questions can eventually lead to talking about the coefficient of friction, to "loose molecular bonding" that causes friction, and so on.

As demonstrated in the ABEL system (discussed below) a similar situation exists in medicine, and one can indeed model causality in medicine at different levels of detail. (ABEL describes it as multiple levels of *abstraction*.) The desire to model a medical problem at multiple levels of detail stems from a number of considerations.

1. For most clinical advice, a fairly superficial level of causality is probably all that need be considered.
2. At the same time, one would like a system to be able to fall back to a more detailed model if necessary, e.g., to explain its advice in enough detail to satisfy a physician who has questions.
3. In addition, there may be times when a particular treatment or coexisting disease interacts with one of the lower levels of the model. In such a situation, the computer may need the more detailed model to appreciate fully the implications of the case.

What Other Types of "Deep Knowledge" Are Possible?

A final question concerns other types of "deep knowledge" beyond causal knowledge that might enhance the power of a medical expert system. This question is discussed later in the chapter.

Research Projects in Medical Causal Modeling

This section describes a number of projects that are exploring the use of causal models in medicine. The systems described are all experimental research prototypes.

CASNET

CASNET,[3] a pioneering project in medical causal modeling, is designed to perform diagnosis in the domain of glaucoma. CASNET is one of the first systems to use multiple levels of detail. As shown in Figure 2.1, observations are linked by causal pathways from a low level description of a particular patient to states in a pathophysiologic plane. These pathophysiologic states are then linked to elements in a plane of disease states. In this way CASNET explores a "bottom-up" analysis for deriving diagnoses from observations using known causal relations. In addition, CASNET is able to predict the likely course of a disease, treated or untreated.

CASNET generates its causal links by calculating a likelihood for each node in all potential causal pathways. This likelihood value is a function of the "confidence" of an observation and of a heuristically derived weight for the associated causal link. In this way, CASNET has compiled into its knowledge base a set of indices that steer the causal pathway generator to the most likely causal links. CASNET uses "threshold values" to de-

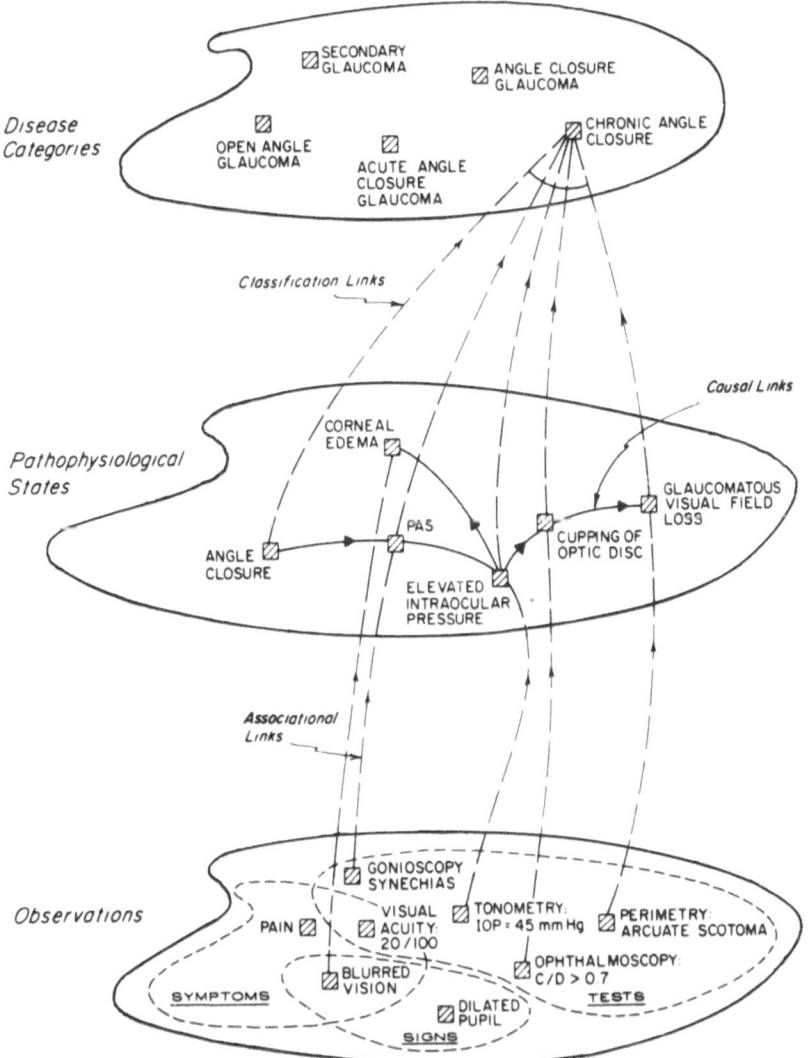

Figure 2.1. Example of CASNET's use of causal relations. (Weiss SM, Kulikowski CA, Amarel S, Safir A: A model-based method for computer-aided medical decision making. Artif Intell 11:145, 1978.)

termine whether a particular node's status is confirmed, denied, or uncertain.

CASNET also explores the use of interactive, directed query. It uses a strategy for selecting questions to ask the clinician based on both diagnostic utility and the cost of a test. Again, this strategy implies that certain goals and tradeoffs have been compiled into the program.

Another feature is a treatment module whose implementation resembles the mapping from the pathophysiologic diagnostic plane to the disease plane. The status of a treatment node is determined from the confidence values of those disease states directly mapped to that treatment node and from predetermined weights assigned to the mapping. Thus CASNET was an early project demonstrating the potential of causal modeling for both medical diagnosis and treatment.

ABEL

The ABEL system[4,5] is designed to offer advice concerning acid-base and electrolyte disorders. The system was specifically developed to explore causal modeling and focuses particularly on modeling causal relations at multiple levels of abstraction.

As illustrated in Figure 2.2, ABEL models its domain at three levels of abstraction (or levels of detail). The highest, simplest level is the clinical level. The lowest, most detailed level is the pathophysiologic level. In between is an intermediate level. Note that certain states (e.g., hypokalemia and metabolic acidosis) are represented on all three levels, as indicated by the dashed vertical lines. Other states are represented on the two lower levels. The causal relations that connect the states on each level are different because they show different levels of detail.

Given a description of a particular patient, ABEL constructs a "patient-specific model" that represents possible causal explanations of the patient's problems at all three levels. ABEL is also able to generate an English-language explanation of the causal relations at any of the three levels of detail.

CHF Advisor

A computer-based congestive heart failure (CHF) advisor[6] is being developed that uses a qualitative model of the cardiovascular system to drive its interactive reasoning. The model is implemented using a truth-maintenance system (TMS) that enforces defined relations between the various parameters of the model. The TMS automatically propagates the effects of a change in one parameter value throughout the rest of the model. It allows the system itself to perturb the model (e.g., by changing one variable) and then to observe how the model as a whole reacts to this change. The system might then undo the change and test alternative perturbations, thereby experimentally evaluating the effects of various therapeutic interventions.

A *diagnostic module* traces causal chains from undesirable effects seeking underlying causes and aggravating factors. A *treatment module* inspects causal chains looking for opportunities for therapeutic interventions.

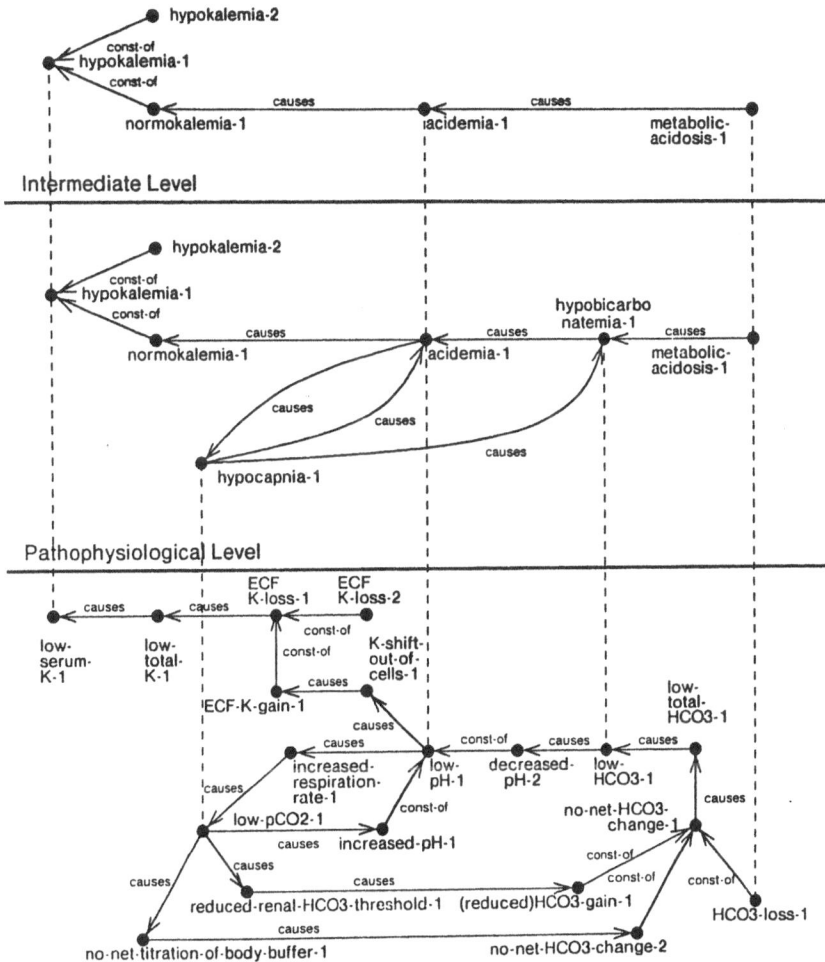

Figure 2.2. Causal relations in the domain of acid–base and electrolyte disorders, modeled in ABEL at multiple levels of detail. (Patel RS: Causal Representation of Patient Illness for Electrolyte and Acid-Base Diagnosis. MIT/LCS/TR-267. Cambridge, MA: MIT Laboratory for Computer Science, 1981.)

To help deal with the problem of interacting forces, the CHF system implements a modification of signal flow analysis, previously used in electronic circuit analysis. The system deals with time by handling the effects of different time delays independently. Specifically, long time constant pathways are assumed to have no effect on the action of short time constant pathways. The system is exploring how such a model could be used to give diagnostic and therapy advice in the management of CHF.

QSIM

QSIM[7] is designed to explore the qualitative simulation of real-world systems and has been applied in domains ranging from a simple spring to the physiology of water balance in man. Whereas one can explicitly solve the differential equations that govern the motion of a spring, in practice it becomes impossible to rigorously solve such equations for all but very simple biologic systems. This problem arises because (1) many of the initial conditions are not precisely known (or knowable), and (2) the causal relations between parameters may be understood only in qualitative terms. For example, if the quantity of water in a man's circulatory system increases from normal, the glomerular filtration rate (GFR) also increases. On the other hand, the exact value of the plasma water volume or of the GFR in a given patient is usually not known.

A key concept in all qualitative simulations is that of landmark values for variables: values at which the qualitative functions change behavior, e.g., a turning point or an equilibrium value. For example, if the GFR can rise only to a certain limit, that maximum value is a landmark value, as is that value of plasma water volume that induces the maximal GFR. QSIM suggests that the simulation itself should be able to readjust certain landmark values dynamically. An example is an oscillating spring whose motion is damped and whose maximum excursion (a landmark value) gradually diminishes.

The QSIM approach has been shown to describe all of the potential behaviors of a system if one takes as a "gold standard" the solution to the parent differential equations, when available. Because QSIM may well describe behaviors that have no real-world counterpart, however, further work constraining its simulation algorithm is needed.

"Semiquantitative" Simulation

Another project[8] is exploring how certain problems inherent in qualitative modeling might be solved by "semiquantitative" simulation. This project uses the techniques of Systems Dynamics, developed for modeling complex systems with many feedback loops. A Systems Dynamics model is defined by "rates," "levels," and "delays," which in turn are modeled by differential equations. Such models have been widely used in management and other domains to simulate the gross behavior of complex systems. The goal in most Systems Dynamics work has been to obtain a rough qualitative "feel" for how a system behaves, rather than to make precise numeric predictions.

These techniques were used to model the cardiovascular system. The model consists of two levels: (1) a qualitative model and (2) an underlying Systems Dynamics model. The system can reason about the qualitative model symbolically but can use the underlying mathematical model to explore its behavior in specific situations. To allow this exploration, the system must first map the values of qualitative variables into "semi-quantitative" terms. Specifically, values such as "normal," "elevated," "high," etc. are mapped into the interval $(-1 \ldots 0 \ldots +1)$, where 0 is "normal." When performing this mapping for all the variables of a model, logical inferencing is needed to make appropriate default assumptions and to create a set of "coherent hypotheses." After the underlying Systems Dynamics model is run, the output of that model must then be translated back into symbolic (qualitative) form by a process of "feature extraction."

This project is interesting in that it proposes a general solution to the problem of conflicting forces by reinjecting mathematics into a qualitative modeling framework. In so doing, it transforms the problem of resolving conflicting forces into the problem of developing an appropriate vocabulary and logic to map from the qualitative level to the underlying "semiquantitative" model and back again.

NESTOR

NESTOR[9] shows one way in which causal knowledge and statistical knowledge can be combined. NESTOR uses causal knowledge to "rescue" Bayes' theorem from its required assumption of independence of antecedents. This work is motivated by a desire to combine the potential power of AI-based techniques (e.g., causal modeling) with the mathematical rigor of statistical approaches (e.g., Bayes' theorem).

NESTOR incorporates the causal links that frequently defeat the straightforward application of Bayes's theorem. Any observations believed to be independent are unaffected. Any observations with known causal or associational links are modeled by causal trees that represent interrelations of the dependent variables. Probability assessments of the interactions between these dependent variables are either assigned or calculated. NESTOR's special contribution to causal reasoning is its use of probability coefficients within a causal tree. In addition, NESTOR incorporates the germinal notion of applying linear programming techniques to solve for probability limits.

Compared to the straightforward use of Bayes theorem, NESTOR has incorporated a causal model of interdependencies. Compared to previous AI systems, e.g., CASNET, NESTOR uses statistically meaningful probabilities, which could potentially be determined from real-world data. In contrast, CASNET, for example, uses heuristically derived weights to represent the "relevance" of a causal link and the "confidence" of its antecedents.

Thus NESTOR breaks new ground by suggesting that causal links can be explicitly represented within a probabilistic system and that such a representation could free Bayesian analysis from its restrictive independence constraint. As an overlay to a straightforward Bayesian system, this approach might improve analytic rigor, and presumably performance, yet be transparent to the final probability inference engine.

RX

RX[10] is a prototype system that utilizes a clinical data base of patients with rheumatologic diseases. RX was developed to explore how a computer system could inspect a clinical data base searching for relations (causal or otherwise) between clinical parameters, e.g., between steroid use and serum cholesterol.

To perform this task, RX requires a great deal of knowledge about statistical methodology that allows it to: (1) propose hypotheses; (2) design a statistical experiment to test those hypotheses; and (3) carry out the experiments on its clinical data base. It creates its hypotheses by looking at a small subset of the data base and then tests them with a larger sample.

An interesting facet of the RX system is that it characterizes the nature of causal relations in several ways. First, each causal relation is represented by a set of features: intensity, frequency, direction, setting, functional form, validity, and evidence. In addition, RX defines the following three properties of causality.

1. *Time precedence.* A presumed cause must precede its presumed effect by an appropriate period of time.
2. *Covariance or association.* The intensity of a presumed cause should be related to the intensity of the presumed effect, e.g., directly, inversely, or according to some other relation.
3. *Nonspuriousness.* The effects should be statistically valid.

In the operation of the RX system, hypothesis generation involves items 1 and 2, and hypothesis testing involves item 3. Thus an explicit analysis of causality is a central component of RX's design.

XPLAIN

XPLAIN[11] implements a novel approach to creating causal models with powerful explanation capabilities. It is generally acknowledged that an expert system must be able to generate robust explanations of its recommendations. Traditionally, expert systems have created explanations using either canned text or routines that translate the encoded medical knowledge base (e.g., if–then rules) into English prose.

XPLAIN takes an "automatic programming" approach to explanation. As a particular system is built, a record of the domain-related design issues is kept, including causal knowledge. For example, if the program logic tested the patient's serum potassium, the system would remember the clinical reason the potassium level was important. This record is later available to help explain the system's internal logic. In this way, knowledge of domain specific design decisions, usually compiled into an expert system's knowledge, is retained within the system and can be explicitly recalled to assist in explanation.

One feature of XPLAIN is the ability to generate explanations at multiple levels of complexity. For example, XPLAIN could offer an overview of its analysis, discuss causal links between observations or states, or explain the choice of analytic strategy.

Do Physicians Reason Using Causal Models? (If So, When?)

The previous section has outlined a number of projects exploring causal modeling in medicine. A more fundamental issue must also be addressed. To what extent will causal models be useful in medicine and for what purposes?

To What Extent Are Causal Mechanisms Known in Medicine?

In certain medical domains the underlying physiologic mechanisms are well understood. Examples of such domains include cardiovascular function and renal physiology. In many if not most domains of medicine, however, underlying mechanisms are unknown or, at best, incomplete and controversial. Thus the applicability of detailed causal models in medicine is bound to be limited. Related questions are the following.

1. Must a domain have completely worked out, unambiguous causal mechanisms for causal models to be helpful in that domain? Might causal models be helpful in a domain where a variety of competing mechanisms have been proposed but none is clearly correct?

2. Even if underlying mechanisms are totally unknown, how might *presumed causal links* be helpful in an expert system's analysis? For example, causal links might be used in a diagnostic system to help reduce complexity in performing differential diagnosis.

Do Physicians Use Causal Models for Routine Patient Care?

There is a growing acknowledgment that physicians do not usually reason from first principles (i.e., from underlying causal models) when taking care of patients. To do so would be to "reinvent the wheel" and would ignore the accumulated clinical experience of years of practice by many physicians. From this accumulated experience, approaches have evolved to the diagnosis and treatment of most diseases. Instead of attempting to recreate an appropriate approach from "scratch," the physician typically draws on this accumulated knowledge. Two ways that such knowledge might be represented in a medical expert system are discussed later in the chapter.

For What Other Purposes Might a Physician Use Causal Models?

Beyond the decision-making involved in routine patient care, are there other purposes for which causal models could be useful? For example, might causal knowledge be useful in complex cases, or when aspects of the patient's presentation violates the normal expectations associated with his disease? Alternatively, causal models might be useful when a physician *explains* why a particular decision was made. (Indeed, a physician might make the correct decision by drawing on accumulated experience but then invoke a spurious or incomplete causal *explanation* as to why the decision makes sense.)

Other "Deep Models" of Medical Knowledge

As discussed in the previous section, the physician may often call on accumulated clinical knowledge for guidance in a patient's care. This section describes two projects that are exploring the use of different types of "deep knowledge" in a medical expert system.

Roundsman: Reasoning from the Clinical Literature

The "deep knowledge" that underlies much of medical practice is the clinical literature. This literature contains detailed clinical studies evaluating the manifestation and outcome of disease and comparing different treatments. A *critical interpretation* of these studies often forms the basis for informed patient care.

In domains where no causal models exist, it is logical that experimental evidence from clinical studies should help guide medical practice. Even when causal mechanisms *are* understood, however, there are frequently different drugs available to accomplish a particular intervention, e.g., to achieve vasodilatation, to increase myocardial contractility. These drugs often have somewhat different clinical properties. They may also have idiosyncratic side effects that are completely unrelated to their desired action. As a result, even when underlying mechanisms are well understood, the clinical literature is still important to help the physician choose among alternative approaches.

Roundsman[12,13] is an experimental computer system that explores how a computer might reason from the experimental evidence contained in the clinical literature in the domain of breast cancer management. Roundsman contains a "library" of knowledge about 24 articles concerning this domain. Given a brief description of a patient and a proposed management plan, Roundsman does the following:

1. It first searches its library for those articles it deems most relevant to the scenario described.
2. For each such article, Roundsman then selects the *patient stratum* and *treatment intervention* that best match the patient and proposed plan.
3. Roundsman then compiles a list of the significant strengths and weaknesses of the study itself, as well as a detailed assessment of the match between that study and the case.
4. Finally, Roundsman produces an English-prose critique discussing the proposed plan from the perspective of the chosen articles.

An interesting finding was that Roundsman requires a great deal of expert knowledge (obtained from an expert oncologist) to perform the various phases of this analysis.

Script-Based Model Involving Multiple Perspectives

As discussed previously, physicians frequently utilize a "distillation" of their own and others' accumulated clinical experience to guide patient care. This process does not, however, involve the purely mechanical "regurgitation" of a completely "canned" approach to a medical problem. Rather, the physician tends to call up a *general* approach. The reasoning process then involves adapting this general approach to a particular case.

The script formalism is an appealing representation for modeling such a general approach. Scripts were originally developed to model the semantics underlying natural language understanding. A script is a temporal sequence of expectations that models, for example, the various steps and expectations involved in eating at a restaurant. Scripts therefore provide a natural medium for modeling expectations and temporal sequences of expectations and for dealing with violations in those expectations. Scripts can also be used to model events from the different perspectives of the various "actors" involved.

An ongoing project,[14] is exploring how scripts can be used to model the evaluation of a solitary pulmonary nodule. This domain is being modeled from *three perspectives:* from the perspective of (1) the disease itself; (2) the cognitive diagnostic process involved; and (3) the actual tests being used. By modeling the domain from these three perspectives, the computer may better be able to recognize whether an anomaly in a case is (1) an unusual manifestation of the disease, (2) an unconventional thought process on the part of the physician, or (3) an unusual use of available tests.

These different *perspectives* on the same medical problem provide an interesting counterpoint to ABEL's use of different *levels of detail.*

Acknowledgments. This work was supported in part by NIH grants R01 LM04336 and T15 LM07056 from the National Library of Medicine and by a grant from the DeCamp Foundation.

References

1. Clancey WJ, Shortliffe EH (eds): Readings in Medical Artificial Intelligence: The First Decade. Reading, MA: Addison-Wesley, 1984.
2. Szolovits P (ed): Artificial Intelligence in Medicine. Boulder, CO: Westview Press, 1982.
3. Weiss SM, Kulikowski CA, Amarel S, Safir A: A model-based method for computer-aided medical decision making. Artif Intell 11:145, 1978.
4. Patil RS, Szolovits P, Schwartz WB: Causal understanding of patient illness in medical diagnosis. p. 893. In: Proceedings of the Seventh International Joint Conference on Artificial Intelligence. Vancouver: 1981.
5. Patil RS: Causal Representation of Patient Illness for Electrolyte and Acid–Base Diagnosis. MIT/LCS/TR-267. Cambridge MA: MIT Laboratory for Computer Science, 1981.
6. Long WJ, Naimi S, Criscitiello MG, Kurzrok S: Reasoning about therapy from a physiologic model. p. 756. In: Proceedings of MEDINFO 86. Washington, DC: 1986.
7. Kuipers B: Qualitative Simulation of Mechanisms. MIT/LCS/TM-274. Cambridge, MA: MIT Laboratory for Computer Science, 1985.
8. Widman LE: Represention method for dynamic causal knowledge using semi-quantitative simulation. p. 180. In: Proceedings of MEDINFO 86. Washington, DC: 1986.
9. Cooper G: NESTOR: A Medical Decision Support System that Integrates Causal, Temporal and Probabilistic Knowledge. PhD thesis. Computer Science, Stanford University, 1984.
10. Blum RL: Computer-assisted design of studies using routine clinical data. Ann Intern Med 104:858, 1986.
11. Swartout WR: Explaining and justifying expert consultation programs. p. 815. In: Proceedings of the Seventh International Joint Conference on Artificial Intelligence. Vancouver: 1981.
12. Rennels GD: A Computational Model of Reasoning from the Clinical Literature. PhD thesis. Medical Information Sciences, Stanford University, 1986.
13. Rennels GD, Shortliffe EH, Stockdale FE, Miller PL: A computational model of reasoning from the clinical literature. Comput Methods Programs Biomed 24:139, 1987.
14. Fisher PR, Miller PL, Swett HA: A script-based representation of medical knowledge involving multiple perspectives. p. 233. In: Proceedings of the American Association of Medical Systems and Informatics Congress-87, San Francisco: 1987.

3
Compiling Causal Knowledge for Diagnostic Reasoning

Ramesh Patil and Oksana Senyk

The use of causality as a pivotal mechanism in diagnostic reasoning was first explored in the CASNET/glaucoma program.[4] The causal knowledge in CASNET is represented as a network of *pathophysiologic states* that correspond to specific physiologic dysfunctions (not complete diseases), a set of *tests* that provide evidence about the likelihood of existence of those states in a given patient, and *causal links* between states, with subjective assessments of the transition probabilities from one state to the next. Each disease is described as a possible pattern of causally related states. Diagnosis is carried out by testing for the existence of individual pathophysiologic states, followed by matching the observed pattern of states against the patterns described for various diseases.

The set of confirmed pathophysiologic nodes and links in CASNET could be viewed as an explanation of the pathophysiology of a patient's illness. In addition, CASNET took into account the temporal progression of a disease and used the notion of causal consistency in its diagnostic process. However, because of the nature of CASNET's problem domain and its limited mechanism for manipulating causal relations, CASNET did not deal with multiple co-occurring disorders. Furthermore, the separation of the process of information-gathering from hypothesis formation prevented CASNET from directing its information-gathering process. Unfortunately, these serious shortcomings prevented the techniques pioneered in CASNET from being applied in a broad medical domain.

In parallel to CASNET other programs, e.g., INTERNIST-I[5] and the Present Illness Program (PIP),[6] were being developed to deal with broad medical domains. These programs were based primarily on probabilistic associations between diseases and their manifestations. As a consequence, they were incapable of recognizing variations in the way a disease can present, both in terms of spectrum of findings and severity. Furthermore, they could not recognize how one disease may influence the presentation of another or how the effects of previous treatment can modify the patient's

From *Proceedings, 11th Symposium on Computer Applications in Medical Care*, pp. 23–29, © 1987, Institute of Electrical and Electronics Engineers, Inc. Reprinted with permission.

illness.[3] It was believed that these problems could be overcome only by the representation and manipulation of explicit descriptions of the patient's illness called *composite hypotheses,* which contain combinations of disease entities and determine interactions among them.

Two efforts were undertaken to explore these issues. The first, CADUCEUS,[7] employed causal knowledge to structure diagnostic problems in the broad domain of internal medicine. The second, ABEL,[8,9] focused on the investigation of methods for dealing with interactions among diseases by using detailed knowledge of pathophysiology within the narrow domain of fluid and electrolyte balance. In the following sections we briefly review the strengths and weaknesses of these two systems. We then present a design for a new system that draws on the proved strengths of each and is further enhanced by a new method for the representation of causal relations.

INTERNIST/CADUCEUS Project

To improve the performance of INTERNIST-I, Pople explored new ways of exploiting the causal relations already present in the program's knowledge base. This study led to the experimental implementation of a new program called INTERNIST-II.[10] This program evoked hypotheses from manifestations in a manner similar to that of INTERNIST-I, but it did not use the partitioning heuristic of INTERNIST-I; rather, it attempted to group the evoked hypotheses into causally related clusters of complementary hypotheses. Unfortunately, it soon became apparent that the exploration of a causal network on a large scale was computationally intractable without more sophisticated representational support and search heuristics.

A substantially more sophisticated use of causal relations in forming composite hypotheses was proposed by Pople in CADUCEUS.[7] The design of CADUCEUS differs from that of INTERNIST in the organization of its knowledge base as well as in its diagnostic algorithm. Whereas INTERNIST used a single hierarchy to represent taxonomic knowledge, CADUCEUS uses a number of hierarchies, each organized around a different conceptual structure, e.g., organ system involvement or etiology. Furthermore, unlike INTERNIST, where the hierarchy was strictly structured as a tree (each disease was related to only one parent of a more general nature), CADUCEUS organizes its hierarchies in lattice structures, allowing each disease in the hierarchy to have one or more parents. The lattice structure solves one of the key problems in the INTERNIST-I knowledge base, permitting a disease such as rheumatic heart disease to be classified as both a rheumatic and a cardiovascular disease.

Superimposed on these taxonomic hierarchies are a number of different types of links that relate nodes within each hierarchy and across different hierarchies. These links form the basis for the synthesis operators[7] defined in CADUCEUS, which efficiently construct composite hypotheses through an appropriate choice of level of disease abstraction and causal constraints. Each such composite hypothesis consists of a collection of diseases, clinical states, and causal relations that attempt to provide a causal explanation of the observed findings. The operators encode the basic premises of diagnostic reasoning: They employ abductive reasoning[11] to embellish existing hypotheses by extending them causally toward their ultimate etiologies; and they attempt to refine a composite hypothesis taxonomically, moving from general to more specific disease descriptions. In the following paragraphs we briefly describe various links used in CADUCEUS and the roles they play in the exploration of composite hypotheses.

Causal links are used in CADUCEUS to represent pathophysiologic relations among nodes in taxonomic hierarchies. When two nodes are connected by a causal link, it is presumed that *every* node subsumed by the cause node can cause *every* node subsumed by the effect node. (It may be viewed as a graphic expression of universal quantification.) Thus causal links that appear between aggregate nodes in the taxonomy provide strong assurance that the refinement of the cause and effect nodes of a causal relation in a composite hypothesis can be carried out independently. One of the major uses of the causal links is for aggregating elements in a differential diagnosis, thereby reducing the apparent number of alternatives to be considered at any one point.

Planning links represent high-level causal associations. A planning link can be used to summarize other planning links and chains of causal links. Unlike causal links, planning links represent possible causal relations; that is, they are existentially quantified over the nodes in the hierarchy. When two nodes are joined by a planning link, *some* of the nodes under the cause node have a direct causal relation to *some* of the nodes under the effect node. The primary purpose of the planning link in the problem formulation process is to allow the formation of causal hypotheses at an abstract level. The refinement of the cause and effect nodes must proceed simultaneously, and only those pairs of nodes below the cause and effect that are consistent with the planning link need be considered.

Spanning links are used to summarize chains of causal links in CADUCEUS.* They provide the basis for the efficient multistep synthesis of nodes that are not causally adjacent to one another. Spanning links thus allow the synthesis operators to limit the scope of their causal search to those nodes that are indexed directly to the node in focus, as any remote node that reasonably could be combined with the focus node is connected to it through a spanning link. Moreover, such links allow the synthesis to proceed even if some of the intermediate nodes (usually clinical states, called "facets" in CADUCEUS) are not directly observable and thus

---

*These links are similiar in spirit to composite links in ABEL.

cannot be confirmed on their own. This mechanism can also be used to introduce additional hypothesized clinical states into a composite hypothesis.

Constrictor relations in CADUCEUS stand for strong associations between observable manifestations (clinical findings) and pathophysiologic states. In the causal network it is often the case that manifestations that do not themselves lead to the final diagnosis may nevertheless permit conclusions concerning intermediate pathophysiologic states. Such "almost pathognomonic" associations are captured in the constrictor links; for example, there is a constrictor link in CADUCEUS from the finding "jaundice" to the state "hyperbilirubinemia." The use of constrictor relations in CADUCEUS is comparable to that of trigger findings in PIP.[6]

A preliminary analysis of CADUCEUS clearly demonstrates the effectiveness of the techniques used when constructing composite hypotheses.* It provides clear evidence supporting our belief that causal relations play an important role in limiting the space of diagnostic hypotheses, particularly when dealing with a complex clinical situation involving multiple simultaneous diagnoses.

Although the composite hypotheses in CASNET and CADUCEUS are similar in form, the capabilities of the two programs differ significantly. For example, whereas CASNET uses a static model, CADUCEUS constructs its composite hypotheses dynamically in response to observed findings. In CASNET the causal relation between two pathophysiologic states is predefined, whereas CADUCEUS is capable of hypothesizing the presence or absence of a causal relation between any two states. As a result, CADUCEUS can construct alternate composite hypotheses providing different causal interpretations of the same set of pathophysiologic states. Finally, CASNET uses a pathophysiologic model that is fixed at a single level of detail, whereas CADUCEUS varies the degree of specificity of clinical states and causal relations to match the specificity of evidence available at any given stage of diagnosis, refining its hypotheses as more evidence becomes available. In the final analysis, however, neither CASNET nor CADUCEUS addresses the problem of interactions among multiple diseases.

ABEL

To explore the issues encountered in reasoning about clinical scenarios that arise from disease interactions, we implemented ABEL,[8,9,12] a program for the domain of acid–base and electrolyte disorders. The medical knowledge in ABEL consists in hierarchic representations of anatomic,

---

*A revised INTERNIST-I knowledge base was used; it is one of the largest knowledge bases used by any diagnostic program.

physiologic, etiologic, and temporal knowledge. The program describes its knowledge of pathophysiology in terms of clinical states and causal relations at multiple levels of detail, from the clinical to the pathophysiologic. The most detailed level deals explicitly with stores of electrolytes in various body compartments and with their movement from one compartment to another. Each state in ABEL contains a number of attributes, e.g., severity and duration. Each link describing a possible causal relation between two nodes (states) also specifies a set of constraints between the attributes of the cause and effect nodes. Finally, each causal relation at a given level is described at the next, more detailed level using a causal network to elaborate its underlying mechanisms. Composite hypotheses in ABEL are described by a set of patient-specific models (PSMs) that attempt to explain all the facts known about a patient. Each of these PSMs is itself a multilevel structure containing descriptions of the same diagnostic hypothesis at levels varying from a clinical summary to the detailed pathophysiologic explanation of the patient's illness.

There are several key differences between the representation of causal relations in ABEL and those used in CADUCEUS and CASNET. In ABEL each causal relation represents a functional constraint between the attributes of the cause and effect states. Furthermore, each aggregate causal link in ABEL is described at several levels of detail. Thus a causal relation that may be captured in a single link at some aggregate level can be described by chains of more primitive relations at more detailed levels.

The critical feature of ABEL is its ability to determine and represent situations where a hypothesis is capable of explaining only part of an observed finding. This capability is achieved through a pair of operators: *component summation* and *component decomposition*. Component summation combines the effects of multiple causes, taking into account possible interactions among them. Component decomposition identifies the components of a finding that have not been accounted for; it is achieved by taking the difference between the attributes of the finding and those predicted by the known and hypothesized diseases in the composite hypothesis. The attributes used by ABEL include, among others, the magnitude and duration of each disease and symptom.

These operators work by translating the interactions perceived at the clinical level to the pathophysiologic level, where they are analyzed; the results are then translated back to the clinical level. The analysis at the pathophysiologic level can be done systematically because it deals primarily with quantitative measures of fluid volumes, total body stores of electrolytes, and so on, all of which can be added and subtracted easily. This mechanism allows the program to account properly for findings in the presence of multiple interacting disorders and to find residual parts of findings that remain to be explained, thereby defining the focus for further diagnostic investigation. Moreover, this mechanism allows us to describe homeostatic processes. In fact, in order to model negative feedback control, which is as important in physiology as it is ubiquitous, one must have some scheme for component summation: the initial disturbance must be combined with the response of the homeostatic mechanism, which acts to minimize the impact of the perturbation on the body.

Attempts to generalize ABEL to broader medical domains present several significant problems. As in INTERNIST-II, the general strategies used for causal reasoning in ABEL are computationally expensive. This problem is especially significant in the case of ABEL, as may be appreciated by considering the cost involved in building ABEL's *diagnostic closures* or *scenarios*. A scenario is constructed by projecting the states of a PSM forward hypothetically, identifying the consequences predicted by these states, with a concomitant backward projection from the unexplained states of the PSM to identify diseases that could account for them. When extending each partially developed composite hypothesis into a scenario, ABEL must search a significant number of causal relations, with each traversal of a causal relation involving predictions about the range of severities and durations that is consistent with the composite hypothesis being projected. In an informal analysis of the efficiency of various components of ABEL, it was found that nearly three-fourths of the time was spent constructing scenarios, with the remainder of the time accounting for all other aspects of model building and diagnostic information-gathering.

In designing ABEL to deal effectively with complex clinical situations, we have built a program that reasons carefully with all cases presented to it, be they simple or complex. The cost incurred running ABEL can be justified for complex cases, but for routine clinical situations this cost would be deemed excessive, as a straightforward case could be solved much more efficiently by a program such as CADUCEUS or INTERNIST.

Thus we are faced with the challenge of developing a program that can deal with a broad domain such as internal medicine, solving routine cases efficiently but increasing the depth of its analysis as cases become more complex. Such a program would use detailed pathophysiologic knowledge, when available, to reason about complex clinical scenarios. We believe that such a challenge can be met by consolidating many of the techniques proved in CADUCEUS and ABEL. Of course, such a synthesis necessarily involves a number of modifications and reorganizations of the existing structures. In the remainder of this chapter we discuss a design for such a system.

Synthesis: A New Design

The salient features of the new system are the following: (1) a principled organization of the taxonomic structures; (2) several types of links to capture possible relations among disease entities and manifestations, ranging from purely syndromic associations to detailed quantitative functional relations; (3) the use of compiled causal links to express clinical pathophysiologic relations and to achieve component summation and decomposition without the use of computationally expensive multiple levels of reasoning.

Organization of Knowledge

At the most basic level, we construct a set of pure hierarchies, each organized around one aspect of medical knowledge, e.g., anatomy, physiology, or etiology.[3] For example, the anatomic knowledge is represented by first identifying entities such as anatomic regions and organ systems. These entities are then organized into hierarchies based on a number of relations, e.g., part-of and contained-in. The physiologic hierarchy begins by identifying various physiologic parameters, e.g., body temperature, blood pressure, and serum electrolytes. These entities are related to one another through physiologic processes (e.g., the process of salt–water regulation controls extracellular fluid volume and serum sodium concentration) that are represented as constraints among parameters.[13,14] These physiologic hierarchies are then used as templates for the systematic construction of pathophysiologic hierarchies, which contain the aberrant states and processes found in various diseases. For example, the salt–water regulation process forms the basis for "errors in the regulation of salt–water balance." Likewise, the organ system hierarchy (based on the part-of relation) is used to form an organ system involvement hierarchy similar to that of CADUCEUS. Each hierarchy so constructed represents one systematic basis for classifying diseases. The final lattice-structured disease hierarchy is a product of all of these dimensions and contains the abnormal states and clinical findings of each disease.

This multistep construction of the medical knowledge base has several advantages. It allows us to represent basic medical knowledge and knowledge about diseases in an integrated fashion. It facilitates the representation of the vast amounts of knowledge required to understand normal and abnormal processes and the respective constraints they impose on physiologic and pathophysiologic entities. Finally, it allows for the principled and efficient implementation of subsumption (Is disease X a refinement of disease Y?), which plays a central role in the process of composite hypothesis refinement.

Relations Among Nodes

The relations that link nodes in the hierarchies can be inherited either universally or existentially, as discussed in connection with CADUCEUS. The axis of inheritance and the use of spanning links is orthogonal to the relations themselves, which reflect the differences in our understanding of the associations among various nodes. Thus we have relations that represent the following types of association, presented here in order of increasing specificity:

Probabilistic: represents a simple association between two nodes without imposing any temporal or causal interpretation; similar to that used in PIP.[6]

Causal association: represents a possible causal relation between two nodes. Can be further augmented by providing numerical measures of frequency and evoking strength, as in CADUCEUS. Such causal relations, of course, contain a weak temporal constraint; that is, a cause must be present before the effect in order for the cause to be an explanation for the effect.

Causal/temporal association: A temporal constraint further defines the relation between cause and effect. For example, a streptococcal infection must precede acute glomerular nephritis in order to be a candidate for its cause, but a streptococcal infection that occurred 5 years ago cannot be considered the primary cause of currently unfolding acute glomerular nephritis.

Functional relation: The relevant attributes of the clinical presentation of an effect, e.g., its severity, duration, and time of presentation (start time), can be computed functionally from the clinical presentation of the cause. These links are similar to the clinical-level causal links in ABEL. Such functional relations allow the program to check whether a given manifestation can be explained fully by a hypothesized cause, but it should be noted that in itself this mechanism is inadequate for reasoning about interactions among multiple causes.

The interaction among multiple disorders is analyzed in ABEL by elaborating the composite hypothesis to the level of quantitative pathophysiology, where such interactions can be expressed and manipulated. This approach suffers from a serious limitation: It requires that each clinical-level causal relation be associated with a specific model of its underlying pathophysiologic processes. When dealing with causal relations between aggregate nodes in the taxonomy, e.g., jaundice and hepatobiliary involvement, the number of possible pathophysiologic processes is so large that such an approach cannot be employed. It is one of the reasons why, despite ABEL's elaborate hierarchy for diseases, much of its causal knowledge is limited to the terminal nodes of this hierarchy. As a result, ABEL is unable to make use of its taxonomic knowledge in the structuring and refinement of composite hypotheses. Without such capability, a program cannot achieve the level of efficiency necessary for dealing with a domain as broad as internal medicine. Furthermore, the important problem of multiple interacting diseases requires that a program support the operations of component summation and decomposition, preferably at more than just the lowest level of its hierarchy. To address these problems, we propose a new approach for the representation of causal knowledge: the use of compiled causal links.

Compiled Causal Relation

Compiled causal links are constructed by compiling physiologic knowledge of the type represented and manipulated explicitly in ABEL. The key to this compilation lies in the decomposition of the relation between cause and effect into two components. First, all the pathways involved in controlling the physiologic parameters used to describe the effect must be identified. Second, the influences of these pathways are determined in each disease in the context of a given patient.

In other words, for each causal relation, a table of clinical parameter values for each pathway is constructed in such a way that the contribution due to each pathway is independent of all other pathways, and the various contributions can be added together to compute the total effect. Thus a general formula is distilled from knowledge about a variety of physiologic mechanisms, obviating the need to encode large numbers of special cases. For example, consider the relation between hypokalemia and diarrhea. The information needed to quantify this relation can be represented by making a table of all the factors that normally influence serum potassium concentration (serum $[K^+]$) and then describing the influence of diarrhea on these parameters.

The factors influencing serum $[K^+]$ and total body stores of potassium can be grouped into three classes: input of potassium, excretion of potassium, and redistribution of potassium between the intracellular and extracellular compartments. Input of potassium occurs through normal dietary intake and/or oral or intravenous potassium supplements. Potassium is excreted through the kidney, gastrointestinal tract, and skin. Finally, the normal equilibrium distribution of potassium between the intracellular and extracellular compartments depends on a number of parameters, e.g., body pH, plasma osmolality, and insulin level. Figure 3.1 shows the factors influencing serum $[K^+]$ that are relevant to the example discussed below. A simplified description of diarrhea showing those aspects that are relevant to the determination of the severity of hypokalemia is presented in Figure 3.2.

Given a patient with a history of 4 days of diarrhea of moderate severity, the expected range of values for the patient's serum $[K^+]$ can be estimated using the above tables. First, using the table associated with diarrhea, we estimate the gastrointestinal potassium loss to be in the range of 60 to 150 mEq/day. Assuming that the patient has a dietary intake of potassium in the normal range and has normal renal function, we can estimate a dietary intake of 50 to 100 mEq/day and renal excretion in the range of 20 mEq/ day to a maximum of the difference between dietary intake and gastrointestinal losses. Thus the overall potassium loss in the patient is estimated

Potassium Intake: ≈ 100 mEq/day under normal dietary conditions. In other situations the information provided in the disease or treatment profile should be used.

Potassium Excretion for Physiologically Intact Pathways:

Pathway	Clinical Context			
	Normal	Hypokalemic	Hypokalemic Na-avid	Hypokalemic Na-avid Alkalemic
Renal	mEq/day	mEq/day	mEq/day	mEq/day
	90% intake ≈ 90	< 20 ≈ 5–20	> 20 ≈ 20–50	> 50 ≈ 50–100
GI	≈10 mEq/day			
Skin	< 5 mEq/day			

For diseased pathways, potassium excretion is determined using the pathophysiology of the diseases involved.

Relation between body stores and serum [K⁺]:

Change in body store per unit change serum [K⁺] in milliequivalents per liter (mEq/l)	
Hypokalemic (deficit)	Hyperkalemic (excess)
200–400 mEq	≈ 200 mEq

Changes in serum [K⁺] due to transcellular redistribution:

	Hyperchloremic acidosis	Alkalosis	. . .
Due to pH	≈ 0.6 m/Eq/l rise per 0.1 pH unit change	≈ 0.4 mEq/l fall per 0.1 pH unit change	. . . .
. . .	. . .	. . .	. . .

Figure 3.1. Factors influencing serum [K⁺] and total body stores of potassium.

to be in the range of 0 to 120 mEq/day. After 4 days the body potassium deficit is expected to be in the range of 0 to 480 mEq, which corresponds to a value of serum [K⁺] in the range of 3 to 4 mEq/l.

Such a tabular representation of the relation between diarrhea and the resulting hypokalemia has the virtue that it can incorporate a variety of clinical presentations. For example, the administration of fluid therapy can be taken into account simply by modifying the estimates of daily intakes. If the urinalysis is available, the estimates of renal losses can be

Clinical presentation: hyperchloremic metabolic acidosis; dehydration; depletion of bicarbonate, potassium, and sodium. Assume normal dietary and water intake unless otherwise specified.

Severity estimation:

Severity	Stool Volume	Electrolytes lost in stool		
		Potassium	Sodium	. . .
mild	1–2 liters/day	10–20 mEq/l	100–140 mEq/l	
moderate	3–5 l/day	20–30 mEq/l	100–140 mEq/l	
severe	> 5 l/day	plateau at 150 mEq/day	100–140 mEq/l	

Figure 3.2. Simplified description of diarrhea.

refined to provide more stringent constraints on the values of serum potassium. Finally, if the patient is suffering from other, concomitant disorders, their influences can be accounted for in a similar manner.

The example above illustrates the compilation and manipulation of a detailed, quantitative physiologic model represented in tabular form. The technique, however, does not depend on the availability of a quantitative model; rather, it has much broader applicability. For example, if the linear decomposition of physiologic mechanisms is inappropriate, a special combination function that takes into account the interactions among pathways can be stored with the table. If the physiologic mechanism is not well understood, but empiric quantitative data are available, the tabular representation can still be used, albeit with some loss of ability to predict the effects of other, intervening causes. When quantitative estimates are unavailable, qualitative knowledge (e.g., the direction of change) can be used to characterize the relations in the table. In summary, the compiled tabular representation of causal links is designed to capture the best available description of clinical pathophysiology, be it quantitative or qualitative, whether based on the detailed understanding of physiologic mechanisms or on empiric observations.

Reasoning with Compiled Causal Relations

Given the rich character of the knowledge encoded in the compiled causal links, the estimation of the functional relation between cause and effect can be made under a variety of circumstances. Such knowledge can be used when evaluating whether an observed value for a clinical parameter is consistent with the other observations in the context of a given case. Thus if all the parameters governing the physiologic pathways relevant to a given clinical parameter are known, the program has only to determine whether the configuration of clinical parameters is consistent with the hypothesized disease process. For example, if all the parameters relevant to the control of serum $[K^+]$, e.g., state of hydration, serum pH, and renal excretion, have been specified, the program can determine if the reported value of serum $[K^+]$ is consistent with these parameters, regardless of the presumed cause of the disturbance. Once this consistency has been established, the system can compare the given parameter values with those expected in the disease process hypothesized to be the cause of the hypokalemia. Note that this approach requires, as a matter of course, that disease and treatment profiles in the knowledge base specify the values of relevant parameters.

If only a subset of the relevant parameters is known, the unknown parameters can be provisionally assigned the values that would be expected for the disease process hypothesized to be the cause of the patient's illness. The effect calculated from this combination of observed and assumed values is then compared with the effect observed clinically. If the match is good, the presumed cause is taken to be consistent with the clinical observations. Otherwise, an additional cause or an altogether different cause or combination of causes must be explored.

Finally, if none of the relevant clinical parameters is known, as is the case in the example above, all of the parameters are assumed to take on the values expected for a given hypothesis. The effect computed from this combination of assumed parameters is compared with the observed effect. If a match is found and the causal link is instantiated in the composite hypothesis, the process of diagnosis can turn to establishing the validity of the assumptions under which the hypothesis was formulated.

Of course, one problem that arises immediately with such a model is that links in different parts of a composite hypothesis may assume disparate values for the same clinical parameter when making predictions. Such inconsistencies would result in anomalous composite hypotheses. This problem can be avoided by associating with each composite hypothesis the assumptions already made in projecting the links present in that composite. Furthermore, each instantiated link maintains dependency pointers into the assumptions data base. A simple truth-maintenance mechanism[15] can then be used to ensure that all causal relations within a single composite hypothesis make consistent assumptions.

This technique of explicitly keeping track of the assumptions under which a composite hypothesis is formulated also provides valuable information for guiding the process of differential diagnosis. For example, if two hypotheses assume different values for a clinical parameter that is not yet known, this parameter may play an important role in differentiating between them. Furthermore, the diagnostic importance of a clinical parameter in a composite hypothesis is directly proportional to the number of links that use it. Such information can be exploited when focusing the information-gathering strategies of the program.

An Example

To illustrate the use of the compiled causal links in the presence of multiple interacting disorders, we consider the assessment of a patient's potassium balance in the presence of diarrhea and vomiting. Recall that the physiologic pathways involved in body potassium regulation and the disease description of diarrhea are shown in Figures 3.1 and 3.2, respectively. Figure 3.3 shows an abbreviated version of the description of vomiting that would be stored in the knowledge base. (The figures and example are based on data and clinical cases presented elsewhere.[16,17])

Let us consider an otherwise healthy adult man who presents after 3 days of severe diarrhea and vomiting with poor food intake. The serum electrolytes on admission are (mEq/l): sodium 136, chloride 100, potassium 2.5, bicarbonate 25. The PCO_2 is 40 and the pH 7.40. In this case, because the pH is normal we may assume that the decrease in serum $[K^+]$ reflects the body K^+ deficit, without any component of transcellular shift of K^+. Thus we calculate an expected deficit of 300 to 600 mEq in body potassium. Next we determine if this value is consistent with the clinical presentation.

During 3 days of severe diarrhea, the patient would be expected to lose about 450 mEq of his body potassium through the lower gastrointestinal tract. Because the pH is normal, the renal pathway loss amounts to about

Clinical presentation: metabolic alkalosis; dehydration; sodium-avidity; depletion of potassium, chloride and sodium; excess of bicarbonate. Assume poor dietary intake and normal water intake unless otherwise specified.

Severity measure: estimated from severity of the metabolic alkalosis.

Severity	Serum electrolyte values		
	Serum Bicarbonate (mEq/l)	Serum Potassium (mEq/l)	. . .
mild	< 30	> 3.5	
moderate	30–40	2.5–3.5	
severe	40–75	1.8–2.5	

Additional information:

Serum bicarbonate: > 50 mEq/l occurs almost exclusively in gastric alkalosis
Gastric juice $[K^+]$: ≈ 10 mEq/l
Urine $[K^+]$: 50–100 mEq/l
Urine $[Cl^-]$: < 10 mEq/l

Figure 3.3. Simplified description of vomiting.

20 mEq K^+ per day, as shown in Figure 3.1 for a hypokalemic, sodium-avid patient. In addition, the patient loses a small amount of K^+ in the vomitus itself, perhaps 15 mEq K^+ per day, if the volume of vomitus is between 1 and 2 l per day. The total expected loss of body K^+ in 3 days is (450 + 60 + 45), or 555 mEq, which is in the range of what we predicted from the serum $[K^+]$ and pH.

To demonstrate the ease with which such a technique can be adapted to different clinical situations, let us consider the situation in which a similar patient presents with a pH in the alkalotic range (i.e., vomiting is the dominant disturbance). In this case the total body K^+ deficit would have been much greater, as an alkalemic, sodium-avid, hypokalemic patient loses 50 to 100 mEqK^+/l via the renal pathway. This urine K^+ loss would be superimposed on the lower gastrointestinal K^+ loss from the diarrhea. An additional small decrease in the serum $[K^+]$ would result from the transcellular shift of K^+ into the cells due to alkalosis. Thus we would expect the value of serum potassium to be somewhat lower than in the case presented above.

Conclusion

We have outlined the design for a diagnostic program currently under development that gives promise of being as efficient as INTERNIST-I or PIP when a case is relatively simple and yet deals with complex clinical cases by using detailed pathophysiologic knowledge. This design is based on the organization of knowledge into multiple hierarchies interconnected by links ranging in specificity from probabilistic associations to functional relations between attributes of cause and effect. In particular, we have presented a new method for describing causal relations by using a compiled tabular representation that captures the best available clinical-level description of physiologic knowledge, whether based on the understanding of detailed, quantified mechanisms or on empiric observations. Moreover, this method is designed to make full use of the hierarchic disease descriptions for the efficient formulation of composite hypotheses. We believe that the further exploration of such techniques is essential to reaching the next plateau of performance in computer-based medical diagnosis.

References

1. Patil RS: Review of causal reasoning in medical diagnosis. p. 11. In: Proceedings of the Tenth Annual Symposium on Computer Applications in Medical Care. IEEE, 1986. Washington, DC.
2. Barnett GO: The computer and clinical judgement. N Engl J Med 307:493, 1982.
3. Schwartz WB, Patil RS, Szolovits P: Artificial intelligence in medicine: where do we stand? N Engl J Med 316:685, 1987.

4. Weiss SM, Kulikowski CA, Amarel S, Safir A: A model-based method for computer-aided medical decision making. Artif Intell 11:145, 1978.
5. Miller RA, Pople HE Jr, Myers JD: Internist-1, an experimental computer-based diagnostic consultant for general internal medicine. N Engl J Med 307:468, 1982.
6. Pauker SG, Gorry GA, Kassirer JP, Schwartz WB: Towards the simulation of clinical cognition: taking a present illness by computer. Am J Med 60:981, 1976.
7. Pople HE Jr: Heuristic methods for imposing structure on ill-structured problems: the structuring of medical diagnostics. p. 119. In Szolovits P (ed): Artificial Intelligence in Medicine. Boulder, CO: Westview Press, 1982.
8. Patil RS, Szolovits P, Schwartz WB: Causal understanding of patient illness in medical diagnosis. p. 893. In: Proceedings of the Seventh International Joint Conference on Artificial Intelligence, 1981. Vancouver, B.C., Canada, publ. IJCAI.
9. Patil RS: Coordinating clinical and pathophysiological reasoning in medical diagnosis. p. 3. In: Proceedings of AAMSI Congress 1986, American Association for Medical Systems and Informatics, 1986. Anaheim, CA.
10. Pople HE Jr: The formation of composite hypotheses in diagnostic problem solving: an exercise in synthetic reasoning. p. 1030. In: Proceedings of the Fifth International Joint Conference on Artificial Intelligence, 1977. MIT, Cambridge, MA publ. by IJCAI.
11. Pople HE, Meyers JD, Miller RA: Dialog: A Model of Diagnostic Logic for Internal Medicine In: Advance Papers of the Fourth International Joint Conference on Artificial Intelligence, 1975. p. 848. Tbilisi, Georgia, USSR; Morgan Kaufmann Publishers, Inc.
12. Patil RS: Causal representation of patient illness for electrolyte and acid-base diagnosis. TR 267. Cambridge, MA: Massachusetts Institute of Technology, Laboratory for Computer Science, 1981.
13. Long WJ: Causal reasoning in a physiological model as a computational paradigm. In: Proceedings of the IEEE Medcomp Conference, 1983.
14. Kuipers B: Qualitative Simulation in Medical Physiology: A Progress Report. TM 280. Cambridge, MA: Massachusetts Institute of Technology, Laboratory for Computer Science, 1985.
15. McAllester DA: Reasoning Utility Package User's Manual. AIM 667. Cambridge, MA: Massachusetts Institute of Technology, Artificial Intelligence Laboratory, 1982.
16. Cohen JJ, Kassirer JP: Acid-Base. Boston: Little, Brown, 1982.
17. Maxwell MH, Kleeman CR, Narins RG: Clinical Disorders of Fluid and Electrolyte Metabolism. 4th Ed. New York: McGraw-Hill, 1987.

4
Development and Use of a Causal Model for Reasoning About Heart Failure

William J. Long, Shapur Naimi,
M.G. Criscitiello, and Robert Jayes

The investigation of causal models as a paradigm of automated reasoning has blossomed. However, there are a wide variety of views of what a causal model is. The causal models that have appeared in the literature range from the qualitative simulation models of Kuipers and Kassirer[1] to the probabilistic organization schemes of Pearl.[2] Investigation of a particular problem of medical diagnosis or management usually leads to the realization that there is some truth in all of the camps. The problem becomes how to cast the various aspects of the problem into the appropriate causal framework and how to integrate the divergent aspects of the problem into a coherent whole.

Our work on the Heart Failure Program is an example of a domain in which different kinds of causal models are appropriate for different facets of the reasoning. The goal of the program is to assist the physician in the diagnosis and management of patients with cardiovascular disease characterized by manifestations of heart failure, i.e., when the disease process makes cardiac output inadequate for the demands of the body. This domain is particularly rich in opportunities to reason from causal models because the disease manifestations are often the result of the compensatory mechanisms of the cardiovascular system. When cardiac output falls, the system alters the capacitance and volume of fluid compartments to increase the heart input pressure (preload) in an attempt to increase ·cardiac output. This increased preload, propagated back to the lungs and venous system, may lead to the pulmonary congestion or peripheral edema clinically recognized as heart failure. Because a number of disease states can produce the same general picture, the determination of the source of the problem in a particular patient fits naturally into a paradigm of causal reasoning, in this case linking causes to observed effects to produce a causal explanation.

Reasoning about the causes or effects of a state involves reasoning about the mechanisms of the cardiovascular system or the pathophysiology

From *Proceedings, 11th Symposium on Computer Applications in Medical Care*, pp. 30–36, © 1987, Institute of Electrical and Electronics Engineers, Inc. Reprinted with permission.

of the diseases. The mechanisms are sufficiently important that we have organized all of the reasoning of the Heart Failure Program around a physiologic model of the cardiovascular system. The model acts as the organizing structure for the reasoning of the various modules. The modules use it as the knowledge base of medical knowledge and as a repository for the conclusions they reach to carry out their function.

Initially, the model is the repository for knowledge about the cardiovascular system. As input data are gathered, the model is used to organize and evaluate that data as evidence for the physiologic state of the patient. The evidence identifies some aspects of the patient's disease state, and the model structure identifies what remains unknown. From the model, the diagnostic module interprets the known states causally as a description of the pathophysiologic mechanisms and uses the gaps to determine the additional data that would be useful. The model also provides structure for reasoning about the likelihood of particular diseases or complications within the constraints of the existing evidence. Once the gaps in the causal disease description have been filled, the model represents the state for explanation, either in words or graphically. Suggestions for appropriate therapy can be generated from the model by tracing the causal chains from the primary causes to the observed manifestations, looking for therapies that have the potential to break those causal chains. The model is then helpful for reasoning about the possible effects of therapies determined by the condition of the patient. As the user returns for further sessions after treating and gathering more information, the model provides a way of organizing the changing state to understand new data in light of the old. Thus the physiologic model functions in a variety of capacities as the reasoning progresses.

In this chapter we discuss the various ways in which causal models are used in the Heart Failure Program and then discuss the development of the part of the causal model used for predicting the changes expected from therapies.

Uses of the Causal Model

There are four distinct ways causal models are used in the Heart Failure Program: reasoning about input evidence, drawing inferences from known states about other states, making predictions about the effect of interventions on parameter values, and using the patterns of state values and other information to do various kinds of reasoning. Each looks at the model from a particular perspective, requires a particular mechanism or mechanisms for reasoning, and places information requirements on the physiologic model.

Because each of these paradigms of causal modeling makes different assumptions about the nature of the parts of the model, it is necessary to establish a common terminology to put the knowledge in the right places and allow the appropriate interactions between modules. The basic entities in the model are parameters, states (of parameters), measures, and measure values. There are also links between the parameters, between the states, between states and measure values, and between measures and measure values. The *parameters* represent physiologic parameters such as cardiac output or degree of sympathetic excitation. The *parameter states* represent qualitatively meaningful value ranges of the parameters, e.g., excessive left atrial pressure or anemia. The *measures* are all of the entities that can be given values directly by the input. The *measure values* are the allowed values or qualitative value ranges of the measures. The links between these entities are repositories for the needed information about their relations.

Input Evidence Interpretation

Each piece of input data provides evidence about the state of the patient. These data are results of complaints, observations, or tests done on the patient—the observable manifestations of underlying pathophysiologic changes in the patient. That is, the parameter states cause particular measure values. Some parameters have direct corresponding measures, e.g., heart rate from pulse rate (or ventricular rate on electrocardiogram). Others have measures that give information only about certain parameter states, may be caused by multiple parameters, or may give a delayed indication. Blood volume only has indirect evidence. Because high blood volume may cause peripheral edema, it could be considered a measure of blood volume. However, edema provides no evidence to differentiate low from normal blood volume; it may be caused by venous disease; and changes in edema can lag changes in blood volume by days. Still, it provides some evidence if appropriately evaluated. Yet other parameters have no direct measurable evidence outside the laboratory.

The reasoning to interpret the input is the inference of causes from effects. In the earlier version of the Heart Failure Program[3], this reasoning was done by procedures attached to the parameter states that interpreted the relevant input data as evidence for the truth of that state. For each state there was a simple procedure, typically a Boolean combination of measure values or a mapping of continuous measures to a degree of belief in the truth or falseness of the parameter state. The parameter state was set to true or false if the evidence was definite. For lesser degrees of belief, the evidence was used for reasoning across multiple parameters, or the user was consulted. Thus the causal relations were contained in the procedures from parameter states to measure values and the inverse was provided as links from each measure to the parameter states for which it provided evidence. An example is the decision whether the left atrial pressure (LAP) is excessive. The program uses the following form to evaluate it:

(range LAP fd 10 fs 12 u 18 ts 25 td)

Thus if the LAP is greater than 25, it is definitely true (td) that it is excessive. If the LAP is between 18 and 25, it is strong evidence (ts) that it is excessive, and so forth. The variation in what is excessive in a patient depends on how long the pressure has been high and the physiologic state of the heart. One problem with this approach is the need to account for the a priori likelihood of each parameter state. One could include clauses in the procedures utilizing evidence about the states of other parameters, but then the locality of the reasoning is soon lost.

The approach we have been developing more recently is to use the notion of Bayesian probabilistic networks for inferring causes.[2] With this formalism, the links from parameter state to measure value include the probability for each direct effect. The causal model specifies the dependencies in the probabilities. The advantage is that the probabilities of the parameters can easily be included in the computations. For example, dyspnea is a symptom that is evidence for pulmonary venous congestion, which can be caused (P+) by high left atrial pressure:

```
(defnode pulmonary-congestion
    causes (P+ ((high la-press) :prob 0.7))
    measure ((dyspnea (prob (or at-rest on-exertion) 0.8))
    ..))
```

Also, a diastolic murmur is evidence for mitral stenosis, which can cause high left atrial pressure. Thus even without having enough evidence to conclude the pulmonary venous congestion or mitral stenosis definitely, there may be strong evidence of high left atrial pressure. The difficulty with this approach is handling loops and rejoins in the network. The computational formalism requires that the network be free of loops. However, as the parameter states acquire values, the network becomes cut and the number of probabilistic computations prevented by rejoins decreases. Although there are still rejoins in the causal relations, we estimate the probabilities. The causal model specifies the pathways over which one event, a cause, can influence the probability of another, the effect.

Propagation of State Information

Once some of the parameter states have been given values, a second kind of causal reasoning takes place. Among the various parameters there are two kinds of constraint implicit in the causal relations. In situations where it is natural to think of a state of a parameter causing a state of another parameter, there are logical constraints depending on the nature of the causal relation. In situations where there are functional constraints among quantitative parameters, there are implications for parameter values as other parameters receive values.

Among parameters with qualitative values, the logical implications of the values depend on the strength and direction of causality and on any time lag between cause and effect. Five types of causality have different logical consequences.

1. If the cause definitely produces the effect (a definite cause), the cause implies the effect.
2. If the cause may produce the effect (a possible cause), the effect implies one or more of the possible or definite causes.
3. If the cause may only precipitate the effect or make it worse, but is insufficient to produce the effect by itself (a worsening factor), the cause–effect time relation may be from the worsening factor to the effect.
4. If the cause definitely eliminates the effect (a definite correction), the correction implies that the effect is false unless a definite cause exists. (If a correction takes precedence over an otherwise definite cause, the logic can be handled by Boolean combinations.)
5. If the cause may eliminate the effect (a possible correction), the correction effect time relation may be from the possible correcting factor to the effect.

These logical consequences of the causal relations are enforced among parameter states by a truth maintenance system[4] (TMS). Thus when a qualitative state is asserted (e.g., by input evidence reasoning), the logical implications of that state are automatically propagated to other states because of the causal relations among states. For example, if something is asserted that has only one cause, the TMS makes the cause true as well, supported by the effect.

The Heart Failure Program also has parameters with quantitative values. The relations between parameters with quantitative values are constraint equations, e.g., the relation between cardiac output (CO), mean arterial pressure (MAP), and systemic vascular resistance (SVR):

$$MAP = CO \times SVR$$

The logical implications of these values are maintained by enforcing the constraint equations whenever enough of the parameter values have been specified to determine the rest. If MAP and CO are known, the SVR is automatically computed and made available to the program.

These two forms of causal reasoning to determine parameter values from other parameter values are handled automatically by the system. However, the justifications for the deductions are maintained to allow explanation, retraction, and reasoning about inconsistencies.

Predicting Intervention Effects

One function of the program is to provide reasonable expectations for the effects of therapies that might benefit the patient. Because therapies perturb the physiologic state of the cardiovascular system, the effects depend on the pathophysiologic state. Therefore a fixed list of therapy effects is insufficient to predict the effects in the individual. The way the program determines effects is to infer them from a constraint model of the relations between parameters. We have experimented with both a qualitative empirically determined constraint model and a quantitative model; we have been better able to account for the effects of the disease states with the quantitative model.

The method we are using to predict effects has been developed from signal flow analysis. Each of the therapies can be viewed as a signal applied to the network of parameters with gains between parameters determined by the equations. The model is then a network of causal pathways from the therapy, the source of the change, to all the other parameters. The change along each pathway is determined by the gains between parameters along that pathway, tempered by the feedback relations encountered by the pathway. The algorithm for determining the change in each parameter is derived from Mason's general gain formula.[5] The implementation maintains a record of the pathways from the change to the other parameters, providing a basis for generating causal explanations for the predictions.

The development of a model for predicting the effects of therapy in the pertinent disease states has been the subject of much of our research over the past year. The challenges and problems of this kind of model development is discussed under Development of the Predictive Model, below.

Constrained Model as Patterns

Once some parameters have states from input evidence and others have values by implication, causal reasoning from the patterns of states can take place. It includes diagnostic reasoning, reasoning about appropriate therapies, tracking changes across multiple sessions, and providing explanations of the reasoning conclusions.

Diagnostic reasoning is the process of inferring from the known states the likely chains of abnormal states from primary causes to observed manifestations. Typically they are "causal trees" with branches added to the primary cause by complications. It is particularly important in this domain to find the complications because the primary disease is often untreatable. For example, although the primary cause for a patient's angina may be fixed obstruction in the coronary arteries, the complication of a rapid heart rate is easily treated and the therapy may delay or eliminate the need for surgery. The diagnostic reasoning includes identifying the causal chains by following links between abnormal states, suggesting measurements when there are unknown states along the causal paths, and filling in gaps. The model is also examined for parameter states needed for patient management, including states that might change the effect of therapy. When additional states need resolution, the diagnostic module searches for appropriate measurements to be given to the user. A final function of the diagnostic module is to suggest reasonable hypotheses for unknown parameters when no more input information is available, e.g., suggesting an intermediate pathway between a state without a determined cause and an earlier state that might have an effect.

Reasoning about therapies from the model requires searching from causes to the observed effects looking for potential corrections. There may be therapies directly on the causal pathway or indirect effects of therapies. This kind of reasoning suggests therapies having the potential to correct the problem or some part of it, but it does not guarantee that the therapy's benefits outweigh other possible detrimental effects. For example, the situation with angina and a rapid heart rate suggests the drug propranolol, because it decreases the heart rate. However, it also decreases the ability of the heart to pump and so may have detrimental effects if the patient has heart failure. Thus it is necessary to include predictive reasoning to determine if the therapy is appropriate under the circumstances.

As the user enters multiple sessions about the patient, it is necessary to relate the new states to the old states. Some of the old states, because of their persistence, provide a starting point for the reasoning in the new sessions (e.g., cardiomegaly lasts for months, at least). Other states help determine the patient's response to therapy and therefore clarify the diagnostic state of the patient. This tracking process is an important function of the program but one that is particularly difficult to understand and replicate algorithmically. Thus far we have spent most of our energies working out the reasoning involved in a single session.

Finally, an important function of the reasoning is explaining and justifying the conclusions. All of the reasoning described leaves justification trails in the model to assist in the explanation process. If the user asks why a parameter state is true, the explanation module can determine whether it was concluded from direct input evidence, by logical implication from some other state, or hypothesized from other considerations in the model. If input evidence determined the state, the user can examine the measures and formula or probabilities that produced that conclusion. Diagnostic conclusions and prediction results are explained from the model structure. The diagnosis explanation simply highlights the states and links in the causal chain to show the user graphically the paths from cause to effect. Each state and link in the presentation is available for more detailed explanation. Predictions of therapy effect are explained by highlighting the pathways that have the strongest effect on that change. This type of

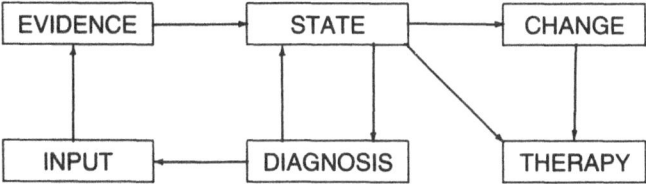

Figure 4.1. Interfaces between reasoning mechanisms.

explanation is useful because it highlights the relations in the model that are most influential in the change.

Interfaces Between Causal Models

Each of these paradigms for causal reasoning assumes a particular uniform view of the domain in which it is reasoning. Within that domain it operates on the information provided and produces conclusions using the subset of medical knowledge provided in the physiologic model for that kind of reasoning. To provide a functional whole, these mechanisms are connected by the objects in the model acting as tokens for reasoning in multiple paradigms. For example, parameter states are both the conclusions of the input reasoning and the atomic facts of the logical formalism for propagating implications among states.

The interactions among the reasoning mechanisms are outlined in Figure 4.1.

Development of the Predictive Model

Each of these causal reasoning aspects of the Heart Failure Program requires appropriate algorithms and medical knowledge base to produce the conclusions needed by the program. In this section we examine the development of the knowledge base for predicting the changes to parameters expected from interventions. Of course, the kinds of knowledge needed and the appropriate representation depend on the algorithm used for doing the prediction. For the purposes of developing the model, the algorithm can be characterized as supporting numerical constraint relations between parameters, including the usual operators such as functional relations, additive and multiplicative combinations, and integrals of parameters. Because the computation is done in terms of pathways from change to parameter, we intend to extend the algorithm to handle relations that are only known approximately by doing the reasoning in terms of limits. Examples of the use of this algorithm for predicting the effects of therapies are given elsewhere.[6,7]

The development of the model was a three-step process: laying out the form of the model, comparing its predictions to reported data from the medical literature, and adjusting the model to correct its predictions.

Form of the Model

The form of the model was determined by the need to account for the physiologic changes that are clinically significant and that differentiate the effects of therapies in different diseases—to capture the therapy effects that might be important when managing patients. Therefore the parameters and relations were chosen for their ability to monitor and account for clinically observable changes. For example, there is a relation between the cardiac output, the resistance through the pulmonary circuit (PVR), and the pressure change between the pulmonary artery (PAP) and the left atrium (LAP). This relation could be modeled at different levels of detail:

1. As a pipe with resistance by assuming a constant resistance for any particular patient and steady flow
2. With variable resistance to account for the decrease in resistance at higher flow rates as more pulmonary vessels open up
3. Modeling the pulsatile flow through the system, relating systolic, diastolic, and mean behavior

The simplest model is insufficient because it does not account for the observable changes in pulmonary resistance in physiologic situations, e.g., exercise. The final model, although more accurate, is poorly understood and difficult to verify because of the lack of available data. Fortunately, the difference between steady flow and pulsatile flow is probably less than 10 percent of the overall effect (inferring from studies on aortic impedance). Therefore we modeled the second view of the pulmonary flow as follows:

$$PAP = LAP + PVR \times RVO$$

$$PVR = \frac{PVR_0 - k_1 \times RVO}{1 - k_2 \times R_x}$$

The pulmonary artery pressure (PAP) is determined by the LAP and the flow from the right ventricle (RVO). The resistance is dependent on the RVO and any drugs that affect the pulmonary vasculature. The combination of therapy and RVO effects is impossible to determine from available data, so this form was chosen because it is consistent with the data and similar to other cardiovascular models.[8]

The overall form of the model is designed to correspond to our normal view of causality. Although constraint equations do not have inherent directionality, people usually think causally in the direction of flow. End-diastolic pressure, compliance, and afterload determine cardiac output rather than the reverse. Because the model needs both the right and left sides of the circulation and each determines the cardiac output, we modeled the mechanism for equalizing the cardiac output as shifting blood volume in and out of the pulmonary circulation. Therefore the difference between the two outputs is the derivative of the pulmonary volume (which then determines LAP).

The minimal requirements for modeling short-term effects in the cardiovascular system in the normal individual include the determinants of output on the left and right sides, blood pressure, sympathetic state, heart rate, and systemic venous state. We started with these relations as expressed in physiology texts and other models, and in some cases derived from patient data in the literature. The pressure and flow relations are fairly obvious at the level of detail needed, so we used relations from the textbooks. The relations for systemic venous volume can be modeled in a number of ways, and the available data for verifying the relations are limited. For such situations we relied on relations developed for other cardiovascular models, usually Coleman and Randall's HUMAN program.[8] The relations involving the sympathetic nervous system are difficult to quantify and have some degree of variability among patients. For those reasons we started with relations used elsewhere and simplified them. It is expected that with these simpler relations the combination of patient variability and missing complexity will be handled as bounds on expected changes. Finally, some relations, including total systolic time as a function of heart rate (not found in any existing models)[9] were estimated from published data.

This minimal model does not include effects of the cardiovascular diseases causing heart failure. We are adding the diseases to the model by adding relations to account for their pathophysiologic behavior. For example, with mitral stenosis it was necessary to introduce a difference between the LAP and the left ventricular end-diastolic pressure (LVEDP), which depends on the fixed orifice of the stenotic mitral valve as well as the diastolic time (when flow occurs) and cardiac output (described by Gorlin's formula). Similarly, aortic regurgitation required the separation of left ventricular output from cardiac output with an additional dependence on blood pressure and diastolic time. At present, we have incorporated mitral stenosis, aortic regurgitation, and aortic stenosis. The model has thus been given its form by using physiologic principles and the requirements for accounting for the physiologic behavior in heart failure.

Comparing Model Predictions

Once the expected relations were included in the model by expert physicians, the next step was to compare the model's predictions to published data. For this test we selected human studies where hemodynamic data were reported before and after a therapeutic intervention or exercise in patients with a defined disease state. There are a number of assumptions and approximations necessary to initialize the model with limited data, appropriately distribute the primary effects of the therapy, and account for discrepancies between the predictions and measurements.

Unfortunately, such clinical studies often report only a subset of the model parameters along with other hemodynamic findings. From these data one must infer the state of all necessary parameters. For example, the first paper we examined[10] reported heart rate (HR), cardiac index (CI), stroke volume index, left ventricular systolic pressure (LVSP), LVEDP, dP/dt max for left and right ventricles, PAP, PA wedge pressure, mitral valve gradient (MVG), and PVR index. The HR, LVEDP, and PAP fit the model, but the other parameters require modification. Wedge pressure was assumed to be LAP. CI and PVR index were converted by assuming a typical body surface area. Converting LVSP to mean arterial pressure (MAP) required assuming a typical pulse pressure at rest and a constant relation between pulse pressure and stroke volume. The MVG data presents a problem of correlation, as the model assumes that MVG is LAP − LVEDP. The gradient actually occurs only during diastole and is more closely related to the mean diastolic pressure in the ventricle. However, regression between the two measures of gradient produces:

$$LAP - LVEDP = 0.808 \, MVG - 4.5 \quad (r = 0.851)$$

This correlation is close enough for clinical purposes. The dP/dt max data did not correlate well with the model's systolic function parameter, but there is no well defined relation between dP/dt max and other measures of ventricular function, so the data were ignored.

From these given data, it is necessary to compute values for the other parameters. To do it we have made a number of assumptions about the resting state of the patient.

1. Right atrial pressure = 0, consistent with absence of heart failure at rest in mitral stenosis.
2. Sympathetic state is set to normal resting state.
3. Reported rest blood pressure and heart rate are actual resting values.
4. Left (LV) and right (RV) ventricular compliance are normal and unchanging.
5. Venous constriction and the venous system are normal.

Given these assumptions, the rest of the parameters are constrained to particular values by the model relations. For example, LV systolic function is determined by LV emptying (corrected for blood pressure), which is determined by LVEDP, LV compliance, and cardiac output. Because the inotropic state implied by the sympathetic state is normal, this value of LV systolic function must be the base value. Similarly, the other parameters are computed from the given parameters. Because of the number of base function parameters in the model, e.g., base blood pressure and blood volume, the problem has always been making appropriate assumptions to give all of the parameters values rather than fitting the data to the parameters, except for such cases as the measured MVG, where something is locally overconstrained.

To predict therapy effects, a model of the therapy is required. As with diseases, these models are being added as we examine studies using the therapies. The primary therapy effects are given in standard reference works, but we have found that the model has sufficient resolution that minor effects often need to be included. We have not found the quantitative information to determine the relative magnitude of these effects or the dosage dependencies. Thus we used averaged patient data from a report to determine the direct effects by examining the changes in the directly affected parameters. For example, our initial model of the effect of propranolol was to decrease the heart rate and inotropic state in the same proportions as sympathetic stimulation increased them. The predictions obtained with this model did not account for all of the actual change in systemic (SVR) and pulmonary (PVR) vascular resistance. A direct increase in these parameters by propranolol is reasonable (and can be found in the literature), because the beta blocker leaves the alpha-mediated restriction of the vessels unopposed (among other effects). When the model of propranolol was augmented to change these parameters directly in accord with the observations, we considered the drug to be appropriately modeled. This modeling process used up two of the comparison parameters for this paper, but important parameters such as filling pressure remain for comparing model fit as well as data on the effect of propranolol and exercise. Because the handful of parameters that tend to be directly affected by therapies have limited interdependence, this approach has proved feasible. Some drug effects are actually on parameters not in the model, so it may be necessary to represent those effects indirectly, but we have not had to face that problem yet. The drug modeling has been done for propranolol, hydralazine, nitroglycerin, nitroprusside, and dobutamine.

We then use the model to predict the changes in all of the parameters, comparing them to the reported changes. The comparisons provide a good measure of model prediction. The problem of model tuning arises when the predictions are different from the reported results. In our first tests of the model, comparing the model to the average patient data in five papers covering the three diseases in the model, there were few significant differences to account for. However, as we have considered individual patient data from the same papers and others, there have been many more differences, and we are beginning to sort them out.

Problems of Model Adjustment

When the predictions of the model disagree with the reported results, there are two possible sources of difference: The data may be inadequate, or the model may be inadequate. Data inadequacies include:

1. Uncontrolled patient state: Anxiety changes sympathetic tone, heart rate, and other parameters. One mitral stenosis patient had an increase in heart rate and blood pressure after propranolol—the opposite of the expected drug effect but consistent with anxiety. Even the averaged data for two resting states in the mitral stenosis experiment protocol had significant differences in some parameters. Also, patients with enlarged ventricles from chronic heart failure may go in and out of functional mitral regurgitation unnoticed or unreported.
2. Measurement constraints: Simultaneous pressure measurements are impossible using the conventional single catheter. Noisy signals and routine estimations also introduce variation.
3. Uncontrolled variables: Experimental conditions may differ from those assumed in the model. A paper reporting effects of hydralazine included 24 hours to optimize dosage—enough time for some fluid accumulation, although the predictions assumed a constant blood volume.
4. Inhomogeneous population: Some papers group patients with significant distinctions together (e.g., different diseases or concurrent therapies), destroying the correspondence between the averages and the model parameters.
5. Recording errors: Sometimes there are inconsistencies in the reported data, making such errors obvious, but most are undetectable.

Except for experimental assumptions, these problems are primarily those of individual data as discrepancies tend to disappear with averaging. A major source of all of these problems is the difference between the experimenter's original purpose and ours. Controls and measurements may not be as carefully done as we would like because they were not necessary to the paper's thesis.

Sources of model inadequacies include:

1. Interpatient variation in physiologic relations: Heart rate response to changes in blood pressure seems to vary in magnitude.
2. Interpatient variation in therapy response: Relative effects of dobutamine on inotropic state versus SVR varies.
3. Unrecognized pathophysiologic relations in disease: With mitral stenosis it was clear that the dependence of PVR on cardiac output was different from that in normals; in fact, the resistance increased at higher cardiac outputs. However, this finding is consistent because many patients with mitral stenosis have had chronically high pulmonary pressures that may lead to permanent changes in pulmonary vessels.
4. Overlooked physiologic relations: We changed the pressure drop across the systemic circulation to be MAP − RAP (right atrial pressure) rather than just MAP because there can be significant changes in RAP in patients with heart failure. We will also have to include LV end-diastolic volume to account for disorders of compliance. The modeling of therapies is an example of handling these factors.

5. Unknown interaction of effects: Two therapy effects on the same parameter may exhibit synergism or interference. Sympathetic tone may alter therapy effects. Such problems are difficult to handle because appropriate experiments are rare.
6. Inadequately modeled relations: One of the more difficult additions is proving to be mitral regurgitation because the changes in the regurgitant volume with therapy do not seem to obey any simple or consistent relation with the other parameters.

The interpatient variations we accept as inherent limitations in the model need rough quantification to give the user an appropriate range of expectations in the predictions. The rest should lead to improvements in the model, although the further down the list the more difficult the problem because of increasing complexity and decreasing data.

The challenge of tuning the model is to appropriately attribute the differences between the predictions and the reported values among these possible explanations. Our approach is as follows:

1. Start with the relations that have been reported and supported by others, as they have been tested by experiments specifically designed to answer the right questions.
2. Where such relations are lacking or are qualitative, use the averaged data reported in papers to suggest simple relations that capture as much of the clinically significant dynamics as possible. The averaged data should be relatively free of errors and inconsistencies and therefore more appropriate for answering questions about relations than the individual data.
3. Sometimes it is possible to find experimental data with enough parameters reported to locally constrain a relation and allow specific questions to be addressed. They need to be exploited whenever possible to verify the empirically based relations in the model.
4. Questions of interpatient variability must be answered with individual patient data. With some care we can eliminate the obvious errors, but the sources of variability will still include both physiologic variability and measurement error. However, that is also the reality when the program is used in clinical settings, so it is not necessary to further separate the sources of error.

Thus with suitable care we believe it is possible to develop a model that will provide useful answers about the likely effects of therapy in a clinical setting.

Acknowledgments. This research was supported by National Institutes of Health grant R01 HL33041 from the National Heart, Lung, and Blood Institute, R24 RR01320 from the Division of Research Resources, and R01 LM04493 from the National Library of Medicine.

References

1. Kuipers B, Kassirer JP: Causal reasoning in medicine: analysis of a protocol. Cognitive Sci 8:363, 1984.
2. Pearl J: Fusion, Propagation, and Structuring in Bayesian Networks. CSD-850022. Los Angeles: University of California at Los Angeles, 1985.
3. Long WJ, Naimi S, Criscitiello MG, Pauker SG, Szolovits P: An aid to physiological reasoning in the management of cardiovascular disease. p. 3. In: 1984 Computers in Cardiology Conference, Salt Lake City, Utah 1984. IEEE Computer Society, Long Beach, CA
4. McAllester DA: Reasoning Utility Package User's Manual, Version One. MIT/AIM-667. Cambridge, MA: MIT, Artificial Intelligence Laboratory, 1982.
5. Mason SJ: Feedback theory—further properties of signal graphs. Proc IRE 44:920, 1956.
6. Long WJ, Naimi S, Criscitiello MG, Kurzrok S: Reasoning about therapy from a physiological model. p. 756. In: Proceedings of MEDINFO 86. Washington, DC: 1986.
7. Long WJ, Naimi S, Criscitiello MG, Jayes R: Using a physiological model for prediction of therapy effects in heart disease. p. 15. In: 1986 Computers in Cardiology Conference. Boston: 1986. IEEE Computer Society, Long Beach, CA
8. Coleman TG, Randall JE: HUMAN: a comprehensive physiological model. Physiologist 26:15, 1983.
9. Brawley RK, Morrow AG: Direct determinations of aortic blood flow in patients with aortic regurgitation. Circulation 35:32, 1967.
10. Giuffrida G, Bonzani G, Betocchi S, Piscione F, Giudice P, Miceli D, Mazza F, Condorelli M. Hemodynamic response to exercise after propranolol in patients with mitral stenosis. Am J Cardiol 44:1076, 1979.

5
Toward the Diagnosis of Medical Causal Models by Semiquantitative Reasoning

Lawrence E. Widman, Yong Bok Lee, and Yoh-Han Pao

The causal modeling approach to medical expert systems has attracted increasing interest.[1] Potential advantages of "deep" causal models, in contrast to "superficial" production rule methods, include truth maintenance, graceful degradation of performance in problems at the periphery of the knowledge base, and flexible explanation.

Two of the central issues in causal modeling are (1) reasoning about degrees of relative influence when multiple forces interact, e.g., feedback relations and competing causal inputs to common variables; and (2) reasoning about temporal information, e.g., time delays. A method based on the combination of symbolic reasoning with dynamic systems engineering has been proposed to address these issues[2] that uses deterministic, semiquantitative numerical simulation in its reasoning method.

A prototype model of the cardiovascular system has been constructed to develop this approach (Fig. 5.1). In overview, the operation of the method is as follows:

1. Observed patient findings are described with semiquantitative precision.
2. Qualitative analysis of the findings is performed to: (1) develop a differential diagnosis of the findings; (2) infer a "consistent set" of initial semiquantitative values for all model variables for each diagnosis in the differential list; and (3) map the semiquantitative value assignments to numbers for a numeric simulation.
3. Simulation of the model is performed for each diagnosis. This simulation is performed after translating the model into a set of first-order differential equations and then integrating them by standard methods. The model is constructed from "building blocks" that describe the functional aspect of the various components in symbolic terms and map directly into differential equations. [In a previous paper[2] this step was described for models that were entirely in the normal state except for perturbations (abnormalities) applied at the start of simulation.]

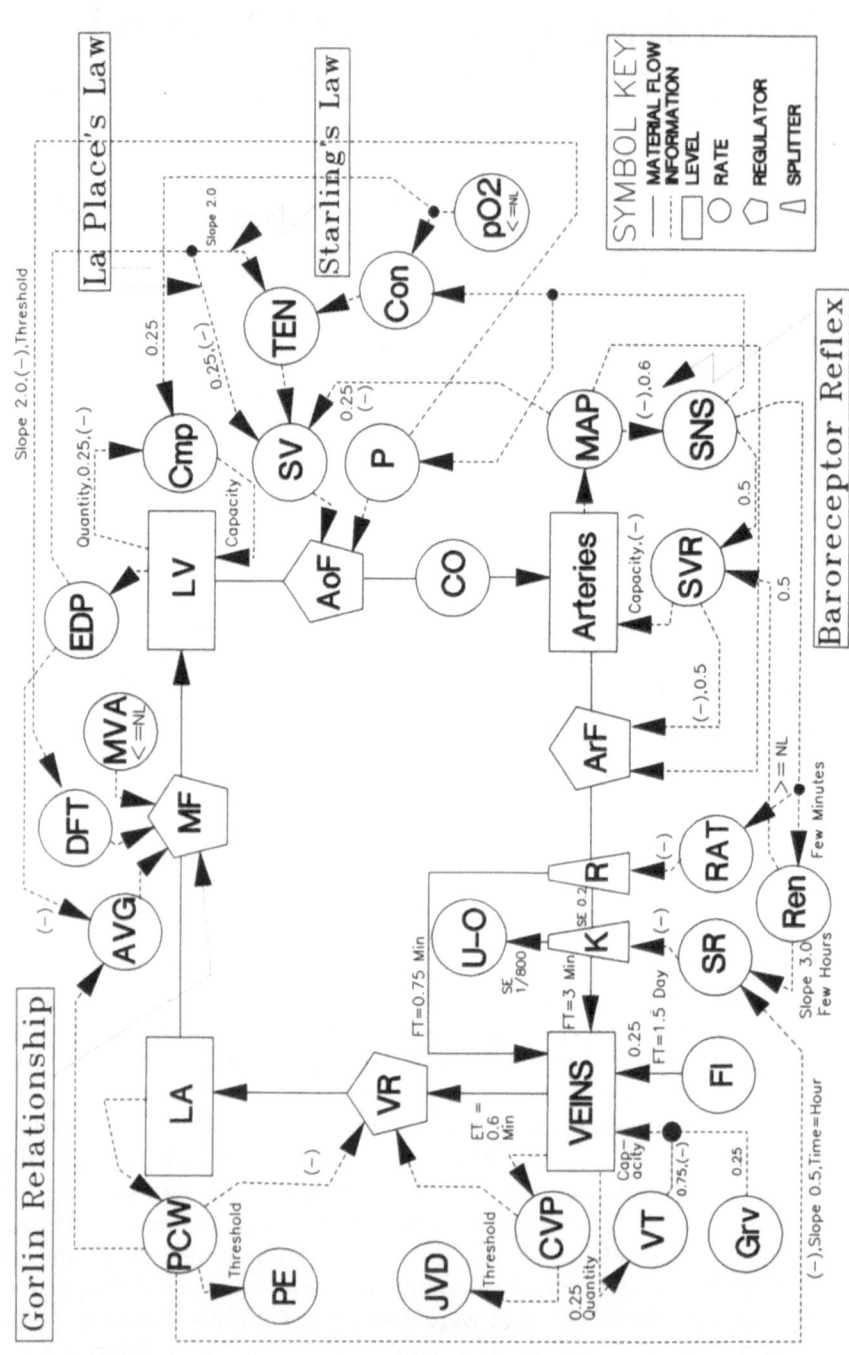

4. The results of the semiquantitative simulation are mapped back to qualitative terms to allow further symbolic reasoning.

The remainder of this chapter focuses primarily on step 2 of this process, the inference of the differential diagnosis and of self-consistent values for each diagnosis.

Definitions and Conventions

Differential Diagnosis

The differential diagnosis is a list of all model faults that could account for a given set of observations. For a typical diagnostic task, some but not all of the model's variables have assigned (i.e., observed) values. The task of differential diagnosis is to identify all known disease states that are consistent with the assigned values.

Specification of Initial Conditions

The specification of initial conditions is a separate but related problem. Identification of the model fault, or diagnosis, is not sufficient to allow simulation of its consequences. Values must first be assigned to all remaining (unspecified) model variables. These values must all be consistent with the hypothesized diagnosis. (A set of initial conditions for a given diagnosis corresponds to Patil's "complete hypothesis"[3] at a single level

◁──

Figure 5.1. Simplified working model of the cardiovascular system. AoF, aortic blood flow; ArF, arterial blood flow; Arteries, systemic arteries; AVG, atrio-ventricular (LA to LV) pressure gradient; Cmp, compliance of left ventricle; CO, cardiac output; Con, contractility of left ventricle; CVP, central venous pressure; DFT, diastolic filling time; EDP, end-diastolic pressure of left ventricle; Fl, fluid intake; Grv, gravity; JVD, jugular venous distension; K, kidneys; LA, left atrium; LV, left ventricle; MAP, mean arterial pressure; MF, mitral valve flow; MVA, mitral valve area; P, pulse; Pcwp, pulmonary capillary wedge pressure; PE, pulmonary edema; pO2, oxygen concentration (partial pressure) in blood; R, renal arteries; RAT, renal artery tone; REN, renin activity; SNS, sympathetic nervous system; SR, salt retention mechanisms; SV, stroke volume; SVR, systemic vascular resistance; TEN, fiber tension in left ventricle; U-O, urine output; VEINS, systemic veins; VR, venous return; VT, venous tone. *Not shown:* myocardial variables. *Not modeled:* right atrium, right ventricle, shunts, valves, pericardium, pulmonary edema-oxygen link, parasympathetic nervous system. *Chamber size ratios:* veins, arteries, left atrium, left ventricle: 20,10,1,1.

of pathophysiologic detail, or the initial-time segment of an "interpreta-tion" of de Kleer and Brown.[4])

Semiquantitative Values

The basic assumption using this approach is that a causal network contains implicit structural-functional information from which the program can make reasonable, self-consistent default assumptions. To allow this as-sumption requires the definition of "central landmark" values and the handling of semiquantitative values.

With this method the central landmark value is "normal." All quantities are therefore defined relative to their own normal values. In fact, all values are ratios of the actual values to "normal" values. Values are expressed as semiquantitative adjectives, e.g., "high," "very low," "therapeutic."

To ensure self-consistency in arithmetic and in representation of user-determined semiquantitative adjectives, the adjectives are mapped onto the real number line. By arbitrary convention, 0 is "normal," -1 is 100% below normal, and $+1$ is 100% above normal. Associated with the mapping is the problem of ranges of certainty. The method uses the mean value of the range for each adjective. Representing "normal" as 0 retains the maximum number of significant digits, minimizing subtractive cancellation error during simulation.

Functional Building Blocks for the Symbolic Model

Variables in the model are parameters of the system being modeled, which at least in principle are measurable. Variables are categorized into model building blocks according to their functional behavior. Each building block can be translated directly into a difference equation.

The two major types of building block are the classic Systems Dynamics categories[5] of *levels* (quantities) and *rates* (flows). With this approach, levels are also associated with *capacity* and *ratio* (of quantity to capacity) properties to facilitate representation of the behavior of containers with elastic walls and the pressures inside them. Other variables include *split-ters*, which act like valves to divide flows, and *regulators*, which act like pumps to fix flow rates according to other variable values.

All model variables are either "material" or "informational." Material variables are conserved quantities, e.g., mass, momentum, or energy. "Informational" variables represent regulatory information or quantities that need not be conserved, e.g., flow rates.

Linkage of Building Blocks to Create a Model

Building blocks are linked together to represent causal relations among variables. The minimum specification for linkages includes direction of causality and arithmetic sign (direct or inverse relation). Additionally, temporal relations, linear quantitative relations, and special parameters for specific variable types may be specified.

Two Nonmedical Examples

This section shows two nonmedical examples to help make the approach clear. These two nonmedical examples were chosen because they illustrate the basic principles of the approach without the complexity of biologic systems.

Example I: Single Feedback Loop

Consider, as an example of a single-loop feedback circuit, the heated house illustrated in Figure 5.2. Figure 5.2A shows a structural diagram and Figure 5.2B a functional schematic. Heat energy is produced by the heater at a rate proportional to the difference between the temperature inside the house and a user-determined set point. Unlike real heaters, which produce thermal energy at a constant rate for a variable length of time, the model heater produces variable heat continuously. Loss of heat energy is modeled as escape through the walls. In accordance with the semiquantitative quantity concept described above, all quantities are represented as a multiple of their "normal" values.

The functional diagram displays *material flow* as a solid line and *control* or *information flow* as a dotted line. *Level variables* are containers of *capacity* C, *integrated quantity* (contents) Q, and *ratio* R of the Q/C ratio.

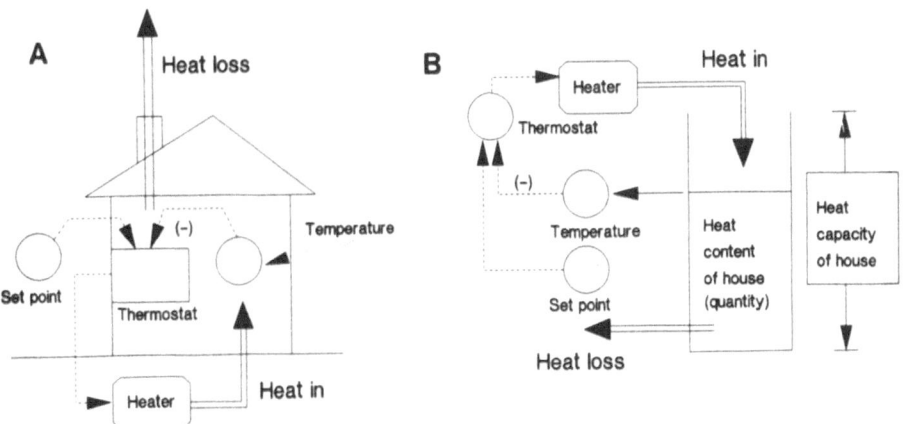

Figure 5.2. Heated house model. (A) Physical structure. (B) Functional structure.

Rates are circles or ovals. *Regulators,* which transform information to material flow, are rectangles with curved corners. A positive value represents flow from a regulator's input material variable to its output material variable. Properties of the linkages, or relations, between variables include *thresholds* and *signs.* For example, using a threshold: if B is a cause of A, B affects A only if it exceeds the given threshold. Signs may be either positive or negative; they are shown only when negative (−).

The diagnostic task can be illustrated as follows. Let the temperature in the house be measured independently of the thermostat and be lower than normal. This condition is represented by a given value of "low" for the ratio in the level variable *heat content of house.* There are now four diagnostic steps to perform: (1) value propagation; (2) hypothesis generation; (3) identification of primary diagnoses or faults; and (4) consistency checking to prune impossible hypotheses. Only after these steps have been performed can a meaningful simulation be performed.

Value Propagation. Inference heuristics recognize the morphology of the graph that describes the model and are similar to the pattern-directed invocation demons of Stallman and Sussman.[6] The inference heuristics interpret the cause-and-effect relations in the model as instantaneous equality constraints among the variables. These constraints are then used to propagate values throughout the network. This step is "constraint propagation" in the sense of Sussman and Steele.[7] In this example, an inference heuristic is applied which states that, "If no variables affect the capacity of a *level* variable, the capacity is normal and the quantity is equal to the ratio." This heuristic is applied to *heat content of house,* which has a constant capacity, to allow the value of *temperature* to be propagated to the quantity of the *heat content of house.* Thus the system concludes that the heat content of the house is "low."

Hypothesis Generation. Hypotheses are generated when ambiguous model contexts exist. Hypothesis heuristics differ from inference heuristics in that they may conclude several values for each variable. They enumerate all possible combinations of value assignments that are consistent with the context. Each such combination yields an independent, parallel hypothesis that is then extended with further inference and hypothesis heuristics until all variable values have been specified or an internal contradiction is found.

As discussed later, the hypothesis heuristics partition the model state space in a binary fashion, yielding a maximum of two hypotheses for each ambiguous context. The use of binary partitioning constrains the search space.[8]

In this example, a hypothesis heuristic is applied which states that, "If the quantity inside a *level* variable is abnormal (e.g., heat content of house is low), there are two possible explanations: the material inflow (a *rate*) may be abnormal (on the same side of normal), or the material outflow (also a *rate*) may be equally abnormal (on the opposite side of normal).

In this example, this heuristic leads to two hypotheses: (1) the inflow of heat *(heater)* may be "low," and (2) the escape of heat *(heat loss)* may be "high." Application of additional inference heuristics propagates the value the variable *heater* to the variables *thermostat* and *temperature*. *Temperature* can also be inferred from the ratio property of *heat content of house*.

Identification of Primary Diagnoses or Faults. Reasoning about the implications of the values of model variables is done during value propagation by inference and hypothesis heuristics. As new values are assigned to model variables, these values are compared *with a tabular knowledge base of known diagnoses or faults,* as in Table 5.1. Each entry in this table contains (1) a diagnostic label (e.g., broken heater); (2) the triggering model variable and value constraint (e.g., *heater* has any value); and (3) an optional list of other model variables and their value constraints that must also be satisfied in order to establish the diagnosis (e.g., value of *heater* has a different sign from that of *thermostat*).

Diagnoses in Table 5-1 are called "primary diagnoses." A secondary diagnosis for failure of a car to start might be "no fuel entering the engine." The primary diagnoses for this observation might include "no fuel in the fuel tank," "blocked fuel line," and "broken fuel pump." Clearly, of course, there can be a hierarchy of "first causes" depending on one's perspective.

In the example, four hypotheses are found (Table 5-2).

1. Assignment of the value "high" to *heat loss* yields a primary diagnosis: "open window." A primary diagnosis having been established, *set point*

Table 5.1. Diagnostic Knowledge Base for Heated House

Diagnosis	Variable	Value	Auxiliary Conditions
Open window	Heat loss	High	None
Closed window	Heat loss	Low	None
Broken heater	Heater	Any	Value not same sign as *thermostat*
Broken thermostat	Thermostat	Any	Value not same sign as *(set point–temperature)*
Low set point	Set point	Low	None
High set point	Set point	High	None

Table 5.2. Complete Hypotheses for Low Temperature

Variable	Hypothesis				Variable observed
	1	2	3	4	
Temperature	Low	Low	Low	Low	Yes
Heater	High	Low	Low	Low	No
Thermostat	High	High	Low	Low	No
Heat loss	High	Normal	Normal	Normal	No
Set point	Normal	Normal	Lower	Normal	No
Diagnosis	Open window	Broken heater	Low set point	Broken thermostat	

must be normal because it can be abnormal only if it is faulty itself. Given that *temperature* is "low," the value of *thermostat* can be inferred to be "high," which determines the value of *heater* to be "high." Thus a consistent set of initial values has been inferred that allows meaningful simulation.

2. Assignment of the value "low" to *heater* yields the primary diagnosis: "broken heater." Because the heater is presumed to be faulty, no inference can be made with respect to the value of *thermostat*. *Set point* is again normal because it is not the primary diagnosis. *Heat loss* is normal for the same reason. Inference from *temperature* yields the value "high" for *thermostat*. The inconsistency that *thermostat* is "high" while *heater* is "low" is permitted because *heater* is "known" to be faulty and therefore unable to respond appropriately to its inputs.

3. An alternative interpretation from the second hypothesis made after assignment of "low" to *heater* allows further reasoning. If *heater* is not the problem, its value can be propagated to *thermostat*. This propagation again yields a diagnosis and an additional hypothesis. The diagnosis is "broken thermostat." The auxiliary condition that *temperature* be less than *set point* is imposed by the consistency check.

4. An alternative interpretation from the third hypothesis with the value "low" for *thermostat* and "low" for *temperature* is that *set point* is "lower," where "lower" is a dynamically generated quantity further from normal than "low" is. It yields the diagnosis "lowered set point."

Pruning Impossible Hypotheses by Consistency Checking. Four hypotheses are thus obtained to explain the observation that temperature is "low." Had further data been available, fewer hypotheses would have been obtained. For example, if *heater* output had been known to be "high," only one diagnosis, "open window," would have been obtained. Had *heater* output been known to be "low" and *set point* to be "normal," two hypotheses would have been obtained. This pruning of the hypotheses is done by consistency checking.

Example II: Two Overlapping and Opposing Feedback Loops

Several more advanced features of the method are illustrated in the system in Figure 5.3, which contains two opposing and overlapping feedback loops. It consists of a pump circulating water around a closed system. The pump output is regulated by four factors: a sensor of the output *(output meter);* a user-controlled rate controller *(user dial);* a protective circuit *(governor),* which counteracts the other two regulators when *rate* exceeds a certain threshold; and the mechanical condition of the pump *(pump condition).* The four are combined in groups of two: *output meter* and *user dial* determine *rate,* and *governor* and *pump condition* determine *pump strength.*

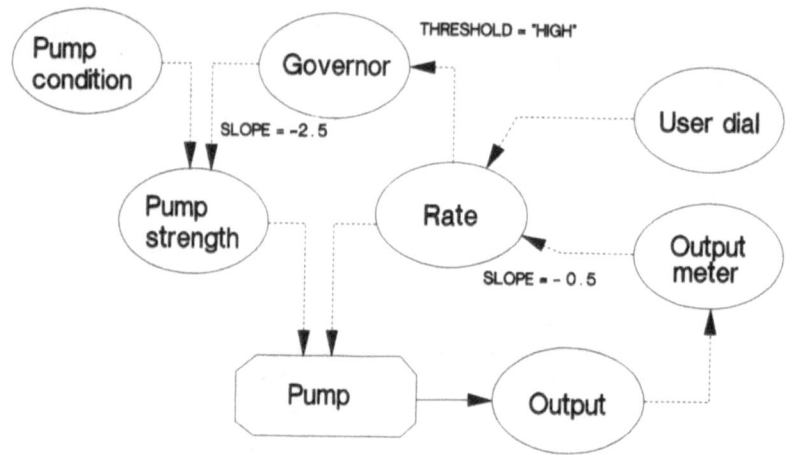

Figure 5.3. Pump with governor model.

The two feedback relations are from *output* to *rate* and from *governor* to *pump strength*. This situation is similar to the combination of cruise control and speed governor in a rented truck, or to abnormal rhythms, muscle function, and the diastolic filling time-pulse relation of the heart.

Consider the condition *output* is "low." If *output* is "low," its contribution to the *rate* is positive, or "high." Let us consider possible causes of a decreased *output*. We can construct a hypothesis heuristic that states, "For each unknown prior variable of a known affected variable, a separate hypothesis can be constructed in which each unknown prior variable is assumed in turn to cause the difference between the known variable's value and the sum of any known prior variables' values. Furthermore, if there exists a feedback relation between the known affected variable and a given unknown prior variable, and if the tentative assigned value is consistent with any constraints along the feedback path, the tentative value can be modified further from normal in a direction that compensates for the abnormality of the known affected variable."

Applying this heuristic, we obtain three good hypotheses and one inconsistent hypothesis:

1. *Pump strength is "low."* This step is an intermediate one that yields two active hypotheses: *pump condition* is "low," and *governor* is "low."

   Pump condition is low. At first, this condition seems to account for low output and results in normal values for all other variables. That is, the *rate* could simply be assigned the value of "normal," as a low pump strength alone accounts for a low output. However, this line of reasoning would neglect the presence of compensating feedback loops. For this reason the feedback adjustment principle is included in the above heuristic. It leads to the conclusion that *rate* is greater than normal but not as great as "high" (the opposite of "low"). Therefore a new quantity, "H-minus," is created to lie between "normal" and "high." This quantity is assigned to *rate*. Given the primary diagnosis of "pump failure," the value "normal" can be assigned to *user dial* and *governor*,

2. *User dial is "high."* Alternatively, one can start with the hypothesis that the influence of *governor* is "low," as an alternative to the previous hypothesis that the *pump condition* is "low." This assertion implies that the *governor* is "high" and allows the inference that the *rate* must be "higher," equal to the sum of the governor threshold, "high," and the value of *governor*. Given that the contribution of *output* to *rate* is only "H-minus," it implies that *rate* has the value "higher," and that *user dial* has the value ("higher" minus "H-minus"), or "high."

3. *Rate is "low."* This statement is not a primary diagnosis but an intermediate step. It generates an inconsistent hypothesis and a consistent hypothesis.

   The *inconsistent hypothesis* is the assignment of "low" to the influence of *output* on *rate*. This assignment requires that *output* be high, which is contrary to the given facts. This line of reasoning can therefore be abandoned.

4. *User dial is "low."* The consistent hypothesis is the assignment of "low" to *user dial*. This diagnosis is a primary one with no feedback relations.

These examples illustrate some of the complex features needed to interface semiquantitative simulation with a symbolic model.

Assumptions

The diagnostic algorithm incorporates several assumptions that allow it to operate efficiently.

1. Single fault assumption. Although an observed derangement may arise from any one of a variety of faults or disorders in the model, it is assumed that no derangement can be produced only by combinations of faults and not by an isolated fault. It is a common assumption for model-based diagnostic programs,[9] although clearly not always an accurate one.

2. Semiquantitative steady state. The model is assumed to be in steady state by two criteria: the sign of the variables and their magnitudes

relative to each other. The absolute magnitudes of the variables, however, are not required to be constant. Thus a capacitor-resistor circuit in which the voltage across the capacitor decays exponentially is in semiquantitative steady state. In contrast, an oscillating capacitor-inductor circuit is not, for the variables change sign over time.

3. Homeostatic mechanisms. When homeostatic mechanisms (feedback relations) exist in the model, it is assumed that they will act to ameliorate any disturbance from equilibrium except when they are part of the model fault which underlies the observed derangement. As in example 2 (above), however, distinguishing positive from negative feedback can be difficult (see ref. 10 for a comprehensive treatment). This assumption can be relaxed but only at the cost of being unable to recognize compensatory changes during backward inference.

4. Quantities and precision of measurement. The nature of semiquantitative quantities is intrinsically unclear: Are they ranges, spanning the set of possibilities for each variable, or are they point quantities whose exact values are unknown? With this method we take the position that they are the latter.

5. Proportionality of levels to rates. A fundamental problem in reasoning about dynamic systems is the lack of an instantaneous relation between instantaneous and integrated quantities. That is, a cup of water may be filling now or may have filled an hour ago: The fact of its having a certain level in it does not make the distinction. This method, for the sake of efficacy, makes the *(ad hoc)* assumption that if the input and output to an integrated quantity are abnormal the integrated quantity is abnormal in proportion, although not necessarily of the same sign.

6. Binary partitioning. The concept underlying the hypothesis heuristics is that the set of all possible abnormal values for an unknown variable can be divided into values greater than normal and values less than normal, and that each abnormality can be considered as a single hypothesis without regard for magnitude. The sole exception to this concept is the case of threshold relations, in which two distinct values with the same sign may be defined by being on either side of the threshold. We have no general proof at this time that this concept captures all possible self-consistent complete hypotheses.

Implementation

The concepts described above have been implemented in Lisp on a PDP-20, in an experimental developmental system. There are currently ten "inference rules" and six "hypothesis rules." The "rules" and reasoning algorithms are still being refined to achieve more flexible and more powerful constraint propagation. Currently, the focus control mechanism is a simple user-controlled depth-first search that allows the user to select which "hypothesis rule" conclusions to apply to the current hypothesis. This mechanism is handy for debugging the "rules" and verifying the correctness of the other algorithms. It will eventually be replaced by an automatic breadth-first algorithm.

Cardiovascular Model

The experimental cardiovascular model with which this method has been developed has 46 variables: four *levels*, four *regulators*, two *splitters*, and 36 *rates* and other instantaneous variables (Fig. 5.1). Note that each level includes two independent subvariables (quantity and capacity), making a total of fifty distinguishable variables in the model. The model has one internal threshold (between *pulse* and *diastolic filling time*), whose effect feeds back into the model, and two external thresholds (to the physical findings *jugular venous distension* and *pulmonary edema*) whose effects do not return into the model. The maximum number of causal prior variables to a given effected variable is five *(veins)*. Most variables have one to three prior causes.

Realistic Example: Complete Hypothesis Specification

Mitral stenosis is an anatomic abnormality found in persons of all ages; it is either a congenital defect or an acquired abnormality (most commonly rheumatic fever). The mitral valve normally prevents blood from reentering the left atrium after it reaches the left ventricle.

When the mitral valve opening is small (stenotic), blood backs up in the left atrium, causing an increased pulmonary capillary wedge pressure (PCWP). At the same time, left ventricular filling is decreased, so that left ventricular end-diastolic pressure (LVEDP) falls. The pressure gradient across the valve, which is equal to PCWP − LVEDP, rises. In the severe case, cardiac output falls, so that blood pressure falls. To compensate, sympathetic nervous system tone increases, causing an increase in heart rate, contractility, and systemic vascular resistance, and a return toward normal of the blood pressure. Thus one would expect that the worst abnormality would be in the mitral valve area variable. The next largest would be in the pressure gradient across the valve. Intermediate would be left atrial emptying and cardiac output because they both benefit from feedback mechanisms. Milder would be the blood pressure, because it starts at an intermediate level owing to decreased cardiac output and is corrected further by the rise in systemic vascular resistance caused by increased sympathetic tone. The urine output, which is largely determined by cardiac output and sympathetic tone, is also mildly decreased.

Comparison of Results Against Simulated Values

A scatter plot of the complete hypothesis for mitral stenosis versus the corresponding values from the semiquantitative simulation algorithm is shown in Figure 5.4. The simulated values, on the abscissa, were reached at steady state in a simulation of the cardiovascular model starting with the assumption of severe mitral stenosis. The symbolic values, on the ordinate, were assigned by the present method of constraint propagation and mathematic relaxation starting with the observation that PCWP is increased and then selecting hypothesis choices that were consistent with the diagnosis of mitral stenosis. Each set of values is expressed as a fraction of the most abnormal value in each set. The Pearson correlation coefficient is 0.89. The correlation coefficient for the diagnosis of congestive heart failure with its steady-state simulation values was 0.88. Although clearly still developmental, this model is a reasonable representation of the human cardiovascular system.

Discussion: Diagnosis in Qualitative Causal Models

The problem of feedback relations has been a persistent difficulty of causal modeling,[8,11] particularly in the case of multiple feedback loops.[12] So far, a general solution to the problem of feedback has not been found. Ap-

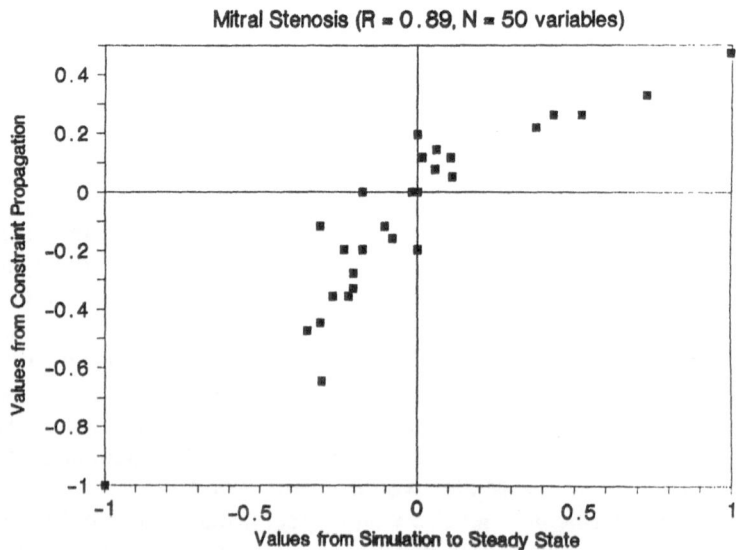

Figure 5.4. Complete hypothesis for mitral stenosis: correlation with steady-state simulated values.

proaches with partial success have included mythical propagation and propagation of disturbances,[4] causal ordering and comparative statics,[11] symbolic propagation with iterative replacement,[8] and heuristics about the structure and properties of equations.[12].

Most research on this problem uses the concept of propagation of constraints.[6,7] With that method, values for a limited number of variables are used to assign values to many or all related variables using the equations that describe the relations among the variables. In some cases it is the constraints themselves that are propagated from variable to variable;[8] in most others it is the values that are propagated.[6] Although propagation of symbolic expressions has been proposed,[13] they are difficult to use in the general case.[8] The use of semiquantitative quantity spaces has not been previously reported, although it has often been suggested.[12]

Simulation using a semiquantitative quantity space is the approach taken here. Algorithms for defining semiquantitative values during the reasoning process have been developed that capture the quantitative differences between actual values by creating intermediate values. Standard pattern-directed domain-independent constraint propagation heuristics are combined with mathematical relaxation to develop semiquantitative diagnoses of causal models and their initial conditions.

The evident complexity of the medical diagnostic process encourages identification of classes of domains within medicine that permit simplifying assumptions. One such class includes those with quantifiable knowledge base variables. Within this class, contributions of individual disease processes can be subtracted from observed abnormalities to reveal unaccounted differences requiring further explanation. This approach, used by ABEL,[3] allows identification of multiple diagnoses with algorithms that make use of the single fault assumption (see above). Although restricted, this class includes many important medical and nonmedical expert domains.

Other problems in diagnosis of causal models include the multiple contribution problem, detection of multiple faults, and reasoning at several levels of detail. If the semiquantitative method can be adapted successfully to a variety of causal models, it may prove useful in approaching these problems as well.

Acknowledgments. This work was supported in part by National Institutes of Health grants R24 RR01320, R01 LM04493, R01 HL33041, 5P41 RR00785, and P41 RR02230. The authors wish to thank Drs. C.C.J. Carpenter, D. Helman, I. Kohane, B. Kuipers, W.J. Long, P. Miller, R. Patil, D. Ransohoff, E. Sacks, P. Szolovits, and M. Wellman, and the nurses and secretaries of the Coronary Care Unit of Hillcrest Hospital, Mayfield Heights, Ohio.

References

1. Miller P: Causal models in medical artificial intelligence. p. 17. In: Proceedings of SCAMC-87 Washington DC, 1987.
2. Widman LE: Representation method for dynamic causal knowledge using semi-quantitative simulation. p. 180. In: Proceedings of MEDINFO 86. Washington, DC: 1986.
3. Patil R: Causal Representation of Patient Illness for Electrolyte and Acid–Base Diagnosis. MIT/LCS/TR-267. Cambridge MA: MIT Laboratory for Computer Science, 1981.
4. De Kleer J, Brown JS: A qualitative physics based on confluences. Artif Intell 24:7, 1984.
5. Forrester JW: Industrial Dynamics. Cambridge MA: MIT Press, 1961.
6. Stallman RM, Sussman GJ: Forward reasoning and dependency-directed backtracking in a system for computer-aided circuit analysis. Artif Intell 9:135, 1977.
7. Sussman GJ, Steele GL Jr: CONSTRAINTS—a language for expressing almost-hierarchical descriptions. Artif Intell 14:1, 1980.
8. De Kleer J, Brown JS: Theories of causal ordering. Artif Intell 29:33, 1986.
9. Davis R: Diagnostic reasoning based on structure and behavior. Artif Intell 24:347, 1984.
10. Long WJ, Naimi S, Criscitiello MG, Kurzrok S: Reasoning about therapy from a physiological model. p. 756. In: Proceedings of MEDINFO 86. Washington, DC: 1986.
11. Iwasaki Y, Simon HA: Causality in device behavior. Artif Intell 29:3, 1986.
12. Williams BC: Qualitative analysis of MOS circuits. Artif Intell 24:281, 1984.
13. Genesereth MR: The use of design descriptors in automated diagnosis. Artif Intell 24:411, 1984.

6
Explaining the Link Between Causal Reasoning and Expert Behavior
William R. Swartout and Stephen W. Smoliar

There is a paradox in causal reasoning. It can be a powerful tool when making a difficult diagnosis[1] and is frequently used when explaining why a particular diagnosis is correct. Diagnosticians in a variety of domains, however, do not seem to use it much when performing routine diagnoses.[2] Why not?

Before this question can be confronted, it is important to recognize that causal reasoning is essentially an *abstraction* of some (usually complex) body of declarative knowledge. In the case of medicine, such knowledge includes domains such as physiology and metabolic processes. The need for abstraction of such knowledge arises from at least two reasons:

1. The amount of knowledge is too great to be systematically searched in the course of "practical" problem-solving.
2. The level of the knowledge is too detailed. Solving even the most elementary problem may involve piecing together an unwieldy number of "basic facts" before one can draw a conclusion.

Reasoning based on causal relations is a form of abstraction that makes such complexity more manageable. We may now reformulate our question by saying: Why is this abstraction often rejected?

One reason is that medical knowledge is not always easily abstracted. In many situations, that knowledge may be too incomplete to admit of abstraction. In others, the knowledge may be so complex in its thoroughness that insights regarding *how* that knowledge may be abstracted are still lacking.

The other reason is that there are alternative abstractions. A major alternative in medicine, as well as other disciplines, is to abstract from the memory of past problem-solving experiences, either personal or acquired from knowledge of case histories. Another is the compilation of problem-solving knowledge based on either first principles or causal relations into easily recalled procedures, e.g., "rules of thumb." Such pro-

From *Proceedings, 11th Symposium on Computer Applications in Medical Care*, pp. 37–42, © 1987, Institute of Electrical and Electronics Engineers, Inc. Reprinted with permission.

cedures may be highly reliable, but the practitioner may not be able to account for why they work.

Part of the appeal of current expert systems technology is that it facilitates the translation of such "rules of thumb" into a working computer program. What these systems lack, however, is any basis for justification for those rules; and whereas we may be willing to accept vague and informal justification from a human expert we know well enough to trust, we are reluctant to put such trust in a software expert and require better justification to instill confidence in any conclusions such a system might draw.

A useful "middle ground" for such justification is provided by the abstraction of causal reasoning. For example, compare Figure 6.1 with Figure 6.2. The explanation in Figure 6.1 illustrates the behavior of an expert system based entirely on "rules of thumb." This system is a digitalis therapy advisor,[3] and in this example it is trying to determine if a patient is abnormally sensitive to digitalis, i.e. might more readily show signs of digitalis toxicity. When the user asks why it wants to know some data, it responds with a brief account of the rules of thumb it is trying to use. This explanation lacks any reference to the causal relations on which the rules are based. Although those relations were known to the system designer, it was not necessary to represent them for the system to *perform* in an expert fashion; hence they were not represented and are unavailable for explanation. Contrast this situation with the account given in Figure 6.2. The same system has now been enhanced with knowledge of causal relations, which allow it to account for its behavior in terms that are much closer to the underlying medical knowledge.

Such causal reasoning can thus be extremely valuable in enhancing the ability of an expert system to explain its own behavior. How can such causal knowledge be integrated with the "rules of thumb" under which most expert systems tend to operate? This is the question we have been exploring.

In the remainder of this chapter we first describe how the XPLAIN framework employed causal relations in the process of designing a routine

---

WHAT IS THE LEVEL OF SERUM CALCIUM?

Enter numerical value: why?

The user types "why?" indicating that he questions why he is being asked to supply the value of serum calcium.

MY TOP GOAL IS TO BEGIN THERAPY. ONE STEP IN DOING THAT IS TO CHECK SENSITIVITIES. I AM NOW TRYING TO CHECK SENSITIVITY DUE TO CALCIUM.

Figure 6-1. A limited justification for a question.

Please enter the value of serum calcium: Why?

The system is anticipating digitalis toxicity. Increased serum calcium causes increased automaticity, which may cause a change to ventricular fibrillation. Increased digitalis also causes increased automaticity. Thus, if the system observes increased serum calcium, it reduces the dose of digitalis due to increased serum calcium.

Please enter the value of serum calcium: 9

Please enter the value of serum potassium: why?

(The system produces a shortened explanation, reflecting the fact that is has already explained several of the causal relations in the previous explanation. Also, because the system remembers that it has already told the user about serum calcium, and because it knows that the same plan was used to generate the code for both serum potassium and serum calcium, it suggests the analogy between the two here.)

The system is anticipating digitalis toxicity. Decreased serum potassium also causes increased automaticity. Thus, (as with increased serum calcium) if the system observes decreased serum potassium, it reduces the dose of digitalis due to decreased serum potassium.

Please enter the value of serum potassium: 3.7

Figure 6-2. An explanation of why serum calcium and potassium are checked produced by XPLAIN.

for dealing with drug sensitivities. We then describe how the Explainable Expert Systems (EES) project has built on those results and allowed us to capture the design of an expert system in a more principled fashion. Version I of EES introduced an explicit representation of the terminology of the problem domain. Version II is concerned with capturing a more explicit representation of the relation between problem-solving knowledge and the underlying facts of the domain.

XPLAIN Framework

The XPLAIN framework[4] and its successor, the EES project at Information Sciences Institute (ISI), have been concerned with creating a framework for expert system development which records the reasoning that underlies the design of an expert system so that better explanations can be provided. With our approach, domain experts and system builders collaborate to construct a high level representation of knowledge of the domain that explicitly distinguishes different kinds of knowledge, e.g., knowledge of how the domain works (of which causal knowledge may be a part), problem-solving knowledge, and knowledge of terminology. An automatic programmer is then used to derive performance-level rules or methods of the sort found in many expert systems from this abstract representation of knowledge. The derivation process is recorded in a machine-readable form, and that recorded trace is used by explanation routines to provide explanations that reflect not only the system's performance level knowledge but also the causal knowledge that it is derived from.

To determine the kinds of knowledge structures that were important to model and what kinds of compilation processes we wanted to capture, we began by determining the kinds of explanations expert systems needed to offer. Using protocols and our own experience as expert system builders and users, we identified approximately a dozen different classes of useful explanations.[5] We used those results to determine the kinds of knowledge structures and compilation processes to model. In this chapter we focus on three types of questions:

1. *Justifications:* questions about the appropriateness of the system's actions.
2. Questions about the *terminology* the system uses.
3. Questions about the *intent* behind the system's goals, i.e., what it means to achieve a goal.

Based on these results, we also identified several kinds of knowledge involved in the creation of expert systems. In our approach to expert system construction, these kinds of knowledge are represented separately and explicitly and then combined by an automatic program writer to create a working expert system. The first two kinds of knowledge we identified were the following.

Domain descriptive knowledge. This is the knowledge that describes how the domain works. In a medical domain it is basically physiologic knowledge, including knowledge of physiologic parameters, diseases, possible interventions, and causal relations among them. This sort of knowledge is that which one typically finds in textbooks. What is missing from domain descriptive knowledge is the "how to" knowledge, which is our second category of knowledge.

Problem-solving knowledge. This supplies knowledge about how tasks (called *goals* in our system) can be accomplished. This category is where knowledge about how to perform a diagnosis or how to administer a drug belongs. In our representation, problem-solving knowledge is organized into plans. Plans have *capability descriptions,* which describe the goals they can achieve. Each plan also has a *method,* which is a sequence of substeps (which may themselves include subgoals) for accomplishing the goal. Capability descriptions are patterns and may include variables that are bound when the capability description is matched against a goal to be achieved.

Our first experiment with this approach was the XPLAIN framework. It provided explicit representations for domain descriptive knowledge and problem-solving knowledge. We used digitalis therapy as a testbed domain when developing XPLAIN. We use an example from this domain here to illustrate how the program writer worked and the kinds of knowledge that were represented. For this domain, the descriptive domain knowledge included causal relations between physiologic states and characterizations of those states:

1. Increased digitalis causes increased automaticity.
2. Decreased serum potassium causes increased automaticity.
3. Increased serum calcium causes increased automaticity.
4. Increased automaticity may cause ventricular fibrillation.
5. Ventricular fibrillation is a dangerous condition.
6. Decreased serum potassium is an observable deviation.
7. Increased serum calcium is an observable deviation.

The problem-solving knowledge consisted of plans (called "domain principles" in XPLAIN) for various tasks such as assessing the patient's state, gathering information about the patient, and compensating the drug dose for sensitivities. As described above, these plans contained capability descriptions* and methods. In XPLAIN, plans also had a third component, called a *domain rationale*, which was a pattern that was matched against the domain descriptive model when the plan was instantiated. Variables in the domain rationale could appear in the steps of the method; and when the steps of the plan were instantiated, the variables were replaced by their bound values.

To illustrate how this worked, consider the plan concerned with the problem of adjusting the dosage for patients who might be abnormally sensitive to digitalis. It expressed the common-sense notion that, if a patient had some condition that might interact with the drug in a dangerous way, then the drug dosage should be reduced. In paraphrased form, the plan was represented as†:

Capability-description: anticipate *drug* toxicity.
Domain-rationale: An *observable deviation* that causes a *dangerous condition* that is also caused by the *drug*.
Method: If the *observable deviation* exists in the patient, then reduce the *drug* dose.

This plan had a capability description stating that it could "anticipate drug toxicity"‡; its domain rationale was a pattern matched against the domain descriptive model to find those cases where some observable deviation caused something dangerous to happen that was also caused by

---

*Somewhat misleadingly, capability descriptions were called "goals" in XPLAIN.
†Pattern variables are in italics.
‡We now believe it would be more appropriate to call this capability "compensate for *drug* sensitivities."

the drug being administered. The plan's method consisted of a single conditional step stating that, if one of the observable deviations mentioned
in the domain rationale existed, the patient's dosage should be reduced.
When this plan was instantiated, there were two matches for the domain
rationale; one for increased serum calcium interacting with digitalis to
lead to ventricular fibrillation, and the other for decreased serum potassium. The program writer instantiated the plan's method twice, once for
each match. The program writer also reasoned about the what should be
done if multiple sensitivities occurred simultaneously (see Swartout[6] for
a description of that reasoning). This entire process was recorded so that
it could later be used for giving much richer explanations that reflected
the causal underpinnings that the expert system was based on, as shown
in Figure 6.2. The critical differences between that explanation and the
one in Figure 6.1 are the second and third sentences of the first explanation,
which provide a causal reason for checking serum calcium. This explanation was produced by paraphrasing the causal relations that matched
the domain rationale of the plan used to generate this code for checking
serum calcium.

EES Version I

Although XPLAIN was capable of offering better explanations, particularly
in the first category of justifications, there were some aspects of its design
that troubled us. A major problem was that the domain rationale appeared
to be unmotivated in the sense that it was difficult to state precisely what
role it played during system creation. Eventually, we realized that the
domain rationale was actually providing an implicit definition of terminology. In the example above, the domain rationale was defining what it
meant for something to be a "sensitivity" i.e., a factor that made the
patient more sensitive to digitalis. We further realized that it was inappropriate to represent terminology as part of problem-solving knowledge;
instead, it should have a separate representation. Such a representation
would also allow us to answer questions about terminology, our second
question category above. When building the first version of EES, we added
terminology as another kind of knowledge to our framework. This explicit
terminology provided us with the building blocks that were used for representing facts as part of domain descriptive knowledge and goals and
methods as part of problem-solving knowledge.

Adding Terminology

In most expert systems, terms and their definitions are understood by the
system builder, but the terms are not explicitly defined within the system
itself. Instead, the terms used by the system implicitly acquire a definition

based on how other knowledge sources in the system react to them and the operational mechanisms for recognizing instances of those terms. This can lead to problems in both explanation and maintenance of an expert system. We wanted to provide an explicit and independent definition for *terminology,* which we defined as follows:

Terminology. This is knowledge of domain concepts and relations which forms the language that knowledge sources within an expert system use to communicate.

To illustrate the problem of implicit terminology briefly, suppose we define a simple rule for recognizing fever:

If the patient's temperature is more than 100°F,
then conclude fever.

Arguably, this rule could be considered a definition of what fever is, i.e., a temperature greater than 100°F. An explanation routine could display the rule whenever a user wanted to know how fever was defined. In fact, that would confuse an operational means for recognizing fever with a definition for it. To see that, consider what might happen if we put our "expert system" out in the field. We might find that we obtain many false-positive results because some people drink hot coffee before taking their temperature. Of course, we can easily fix that by modifying the rule:

If the patient's temperature is more than 100°F
and the patient has not recently drunk coffee,
then conclude fever.

Unfortunately, if we now display this rule as a definition for what fever means, the definition of fever appears to have something to do with whether coffee has been consumed. The point is that an explicit definition for terminology is needed that is separate from the operational means for recognizing when some condition holds.

To provide an explicit representation for terminology, we have been using a knowledge representation system based on the ideas pioneered in KL-ONE.[7] Our representation is based on concepts (which correspond to terms) and attributes arranged in a generalization hierarchy. As new terms are introduced, their position in this hierarchy is determined by an automatic classification facility. Because plan capabilities and goals are represented as concepts in this formalism, the generalization hierarchy of terms induces a generalization hierarchy of plans.

Taking this approach, it becomes clear that XPLAIN's domain rationale was a poor mechanism for dealing with terminology, first because it does not give an explicit definition for a term, and second because it confounds knowledge of terminology with problem-solving knowledge. Knowledge of terminology should be shared across problem-solving knowledge, not embedded as part of it. For example, in the context of the digitalis advisor, the pattern in the domain rationale of the plan for dealing with digitalis sensitivities should be removed from that plan and placed in the terminologic base as a definition for the term "sensitivity." That provides a better representation for terminology but leaves open the question of exactly how that terminology gets used during the program-writing process. At least a partial answer to that question came from addressing another limitation of XPLAIN and providing EES version I with a program writer capable of reformulating goals.

Adding Reformulations

A second problem was that the power of the program writer itself was limited. Although XPLAIN allowed a system builder to express the capabilities of a plan as a pattern that included variables, if a goal was posted and no matching plan could be found for it the program writer was stuck. It had no capability to reformulate such a goal into a goal or set of goals for which plans could be found. We decided to add such a capability because we anticipated that it would provide several benefits. Maintenance and initial system construction would be easier because the program writer would be able to bridge larger gaps between plans and goals, and knowledge would be reusable in a larger range of situations. As we describe below, an additional benefit was that the reformulation capability together with an explicit representation of terminology allowed us to give a more explicit account of some of the implicit operations in XPLAIN.

We identified several kinds of reformulation (see Neches et al.[8] for a detailed discussion). The reformulation we focus on here is a special case of *reformulation into cases,* i.e., reformulating a goal of an action to be performed over a set of objects into a set of goals where the action is performed on individual elements of the original set of objects. This is a kind of reformulation that takes place frequently (but implicitly) in expert systems.

For example, in many diagnostic systems a problem that arises is to determine how likely it is that a patient has some disease based on its signs and symptoms. In conventional expert systems, that goal is usually not explicitly represented in the system because the system designer mentally reformulates it while constructing the system. What does appear is the result of the reformulation: a set of goals that inquire about each of the symptoms individually and a combining function that deals with the problem of how to combine the individual assessments of signs and symptoms into an appropriate overall assessment for the disease. EES allowed us to represent the original goal, the reformulation, and the result of the reformulation explicitly.

We also realized that XPLAIN had been implicitly reformulating goals.

For example, in the plan for dealing with drug sensitivities described above, the capability description of the plan stated that the plan could deal with compensating for all sensitivities, but the method of the plan could compensate only for individual sensitivities. Clearly, some implicit reformulation was taking place.

If we wanted to reimplement the digitalis advisor using EES,* we would model the reformulation more explicitly. The problem-solving knowledge would consist of a plan whose capability description stated that it could "compensate for *a* drug sensitivity." The plan's method would be similar to the method of the plan in XPLAIN. The term "drug sensitivity" would be defined explicitly as an observable deviation that caused something dangerous that was also caused by the drug. When the goal of compensating for digitalis sensitivities was posted, the program writer would find that no plans existed for dealing with sets of sensitivities, so it would be necessary to reformulate the goal into a set of goals over individual sensitivities. Using the definition of sensitivity together with the domain descriptive knowledge above, the programmer would find that increased serum calcium and decreased serum potassium were individual sensitivities, so the original goal of compensating for digitalis sensitivities would be reformulated into two goals:

1. Compensate for increased serum calcium.
2. Compensate for decreased serum potassium.

These goals could then be implemented by the plan for an individual sensitivity.

We believe that this approach captures the program-writing process more explicitly than XPLAIN, and it allows us to capture the knowledge needed to answer additional kinds of questions, e.g., questions about terminology. We also believe that it gives a good account for one of the ways causal knowledge is compiled into expert systems:

Causal knowledge, together with knowledge of terminology, is used during goal reformulation.

In the remainder of the chapter we describe our efforts to capture the knowledge needed to answer the third type of question listed above, questions about the intent of goals. This investigation led us to discover another way in which causal knowledge can be compiled into expert systems.

---

*We did not actually carry out this reimplementation in EES version I. Certain limitations on the expressive power of the terminology representation of version I would have made it difficult to represent terms involving transitive relations, e.g., sensitivity. We are currently in the process of carrying out the reimplementation of portions of the digitalis advisor using a more expressive knowledge representation.

EES Version II

Although version I of EES allowed us to represent terminology and model reformulation, there were two open issues we wanted to address. First, we wanted to be able to represent the *intent* behind a goal. For example, it was not possible to answer the question: "What does it mean to administer digitalis?" Problem-solving knowledge of *how* to give digitalis could be retrieved, but it was not represented anywhere that the problem of digitalis administration was a problem of producing satisfactory therapeutic results subject to the constraint of avoiding (or minimizing) toxic effects.

For another example, consider an expert system we built in EES version I for diagnosing space telemetry systems. This system had several methods for diagnosis, which we have hand-paraphrased in Figure 6.3. They display what the system does when performing a diagnosis, but it takes considerable deductive effort on the part of the user to figure out what a diagnosis amounts to. What we want is an explicit representation of the intent behind the goal in this domain that would allow us to answer: "To diagnose a decomposable system means to find a primitive subcomponent of the sys-

To diagnose a decomposable system,
  If there is a fault in the system,
    then locate the cause of the fault within the system

To diagnose a primitive system,
  If the system is faulty,
    then conclude it is the diagnosis

To locate the cause of a fault within a system that
is loosely coupled,
    Diagnose the subcomponents of the system

To locate the cause of a fault within a system that
is tightly coupled,
  Locate the cause of the fault along the signal-path
    beginning at the system-input and ending at the
    system-output.

To locate the cause of a fault beginning at system 1 and
ending at system 2,
  If system 1 is faulty
  then diagnose system 1
    else locate the cause of the fault along the
      signal-path beginning at the system that system 1
      outputs to and ending at system 2.

Figure 6-3. Methods as an inadequate explanation of the goal of diagnosis.

tem that is faulty." In general, expert systems lack any such specification of what their goals mean. The problem is directly analogous to the problem of implicit terminology cited above. Goals acquire their meaning based solely on the methods that claim to implement them. What we want is a separate definition for goals that users could use as an independent criterion when deciding if the system's goals met their own and if its methods were appropriate for achieving those goals.

The second issue we wanted to address was to better understand the source of problem-solving knowledge. Although both XPLAIN and version I of EES allowed a system builder to represent problem-solving knowledge at a more abstract level than is possible in most expert system frameworks, it was clear that even those methods were compiled from some still more basic representations of knowledge. By understanding the "roots" of problem-solving knowledge, we could provide better explanations of how the plans worked.

Below, we describe the approach we adopted, which is to represent goal intent in terms of a small number of primitive actions and then to mechanically derive plans for achieving those goals by transforming definitions and axioms in the domain descriptive knowledge into plans. We have been exploring this approach in the context of a nonmedical domain, i.e., diagnosis of digital circuits, but we expect the approach to carry over into medical domains and are currently starting to reimplement portions of the digitalis advisor using this approach. Most of the examples in the remainder of the chapter are drawn from our work with digital circuits, but we also outline some of the issues the medical domain is raising.

Capturing Intent

To capture intent we begin by defining a set of primitive actions—actions that are assumed to be readily understood by users. All higher level goals are ultimately defined in terms of these primitive actions. So far we have identified four primitive actions:

1. *Determine-whether:* establishes the truth of a given assertion
2. *Find:* finds an object that matches a given description
3. *Achieve:* achieves a particular state
4. *Avoid:* the counterpart of achieve; ensures that a particular state does *not* occur

We believe that this set of actions will grow somewhat as we gain more experience with this approach. We used the first two actions extensively in our system for diagnosing digital circuits. Interestingly, those actions correspond to the kinds of problems analyzed by Polya[9]: problems to prove and problems to find. We have found the last two actions to be useful in the analysis of the digitalis therapy advisor, as much of digitalis therapy is concerned with achieving a therapeutic effect while avoiding toxicity.

Given these primitive actions, capturing the intent behind a domain level goal then involves linking that goal to its definition in terms of primitive actions. Thus we would define the goal:

Diagnose decomposable digital system **s**

as the problem:

Finding a primitive system **p** such that **p** is a subcomponent of **s** and **p** is faulty

Sources of Problem-Solving Knowledge

The primitive actions allow us to capture the intent behind goals, but the issue remains of how to implement the plans for realizing those goals. In EES version II, plans enter the knowledge base in two ways.

Mechanically Derived Plans. The first way is that plans for performing primitive actions are mechanically derived by performing transformations on the assertions and definitions in the domain descriptive knowledge base. For a simple example: if the knowledge base contains the assertion that "A exists if and only if B exists," it is possible to derive a plan that determines if B exists by checking for the presence of A. Because the implication is two-way, it is also possible to derive another plan for checking for the existence of A by checking for B.* Considerably more complex examples can be handled. When constructing the digital circuit diagnoser, the domain descriptive model was a functional description of the interconnections within the circuit and the functional behavior of the devices in the circuit. Given that description, it was possible to mechanically derive a set of procedures for *finding* the expected signal value along any connector in the circuit given a particular set of input values.

An interesting observation is emerging from our initial work in the digitalis domain: Different primitive actions seem to involve transformations over different kinds of domain descriptive knowledge. The transformations for deriving plans for performing *find* actions involve sets and instances, *determine-whether* involves implications and types, and *achieve* and *avoid* involve states, state transitions, and causality. Thus we are finding that another way that mechanistic descriptions or causal relations can be compiled into an expert system is by:

Direct translation into methods for performing primitive actions

Weak Methods. The other way that plans can enter the knowledge base is by being entered by hand. That may be obvious, but there is one category

---

*Of course, care must be taken when interpreting such plans to avoid circular reasoning chains.

of such plans that deserves special attention. We call these plans *weak methods*. They are general plans, not specific to any domain, that provide a means to achieve the primitive actions in some general circumstances. For example, one of our weak methods involving *determine-whether* states that the problem of determining the truth of a conjunction of two assertions can be performed by determining the truth of each assertion in turn and combining the results in the obvious way. Another weak method for finding an object that matches a description is the classic *generate-and-test*.

Our view of weak methods differs from previous ones, such as that of Laird and Newell.[10] Such views regard the weak methods themselves as primitive elements and problem-solving as the application of operators within a problem space. The alternative view we propose is to regard problem-solving in terms of a foundation of primitive actions that are the primitive elements. Weak methods, then, are concerned with providing general ways for achieving those actions.

Our experience with the second version of EES is still in the early stages. Nevertheless, it appears to provide some of the additional knowledge structures we need to answer our third category of question, i.e., questions about intent.

Status

XPLAIN and EES version I have been implemented and used to construct demonstration-sized expert systems in medical and nonmedical domains. We have tested EES version II on the problem of locating a faulty component in a digital circuit and are now engaged in using it to reimplement portions of the digitalis advisor. An explanation facility was implemented for XPLAIN, and we are currently constructing one for EES.

Summary

We have argued that even though experts may not use causal reasoning, such reasoning is a useful abstraction that underlies many of their decisions. We also asserted that causal reasoning must be accessible to provide good explanations and therefore warrants explicit representation in an expert system. We described three systems that have pursued the explicit representation of causal knowledge, the application of that knowledge to problem-solving, and the use of that knowledge to explain problem-solving behavior.

Acknowledgments. The research described here was supported by DARPA grant MDA 903-81-C-0335 and National Institutes of Health grant 1 P01 LM 03374-01 from the National Library of Medicine.

References

1. Patil R: Causal Representation of Patient Illness for Electrolyte and Acid-Base Diagnosis, PhD thesis, Massachusetts Institute of Technology, 1981 (available as MIT/LCS/TR-267).
2. Johnson PJ, Moen JB: Garden Path Errors in Diagnostic Reasoning. New York: Springer Verlag, 1987.
3. Swartout WR: A Digitalis Therapy Advisor with Explanations. TR-176. Cambridge, MA: Massachusetts Institute Technology, Technical Report Laboratory for Computer Science, 1977.
4. Swartout W: XPLAIN: a system for creating and explaining expert consulting systems. Artif Intell 21: 285, 1983.
5. Swartout W: Knowledge needed for expert system explanation. Future Comput Syst 1(2), 1986, 99–114.
6. Swartout W: Producing Explanations and Justifications of Expert Consulting Systems. Technical Report 251. Cambridge, MA: MIT, 1981.
7. Brachman R: A Structural Paradigm for Representing Knowledge. Report No. 3605. Cambridge, MA: Bolt, Beranek & Newman, 1978.
8. Neches R, Swartout WR, and Moore JD: Enhanced maintenance and explanation of expert systems through explicit models of their development. IEEE Transactions on Software Engineering SE-11, (11), November 1985, 1337–1351.
9. Polya G: How To Solve It: A New Aspect of Mathematical Method. 2nd Ed. Princeton: Princeton University Press, 1971.
10. Laird J, Newell A: A Universal Weak Method. Technical Report CMU-CS-83-141. Pittsburgh: Carnegie-Mellon University Department of Computer Science, 1983.

7
Computer-Based Medical Diagnosis Using Belief Networks and Bounded Probabilities

Gregory F. Cooper

Accurate diagnosis is of central importance for good medical decision-making. Diagnosis can be complex, however, particularly as the amount of general medical knowledge accumulates and as patients become more medically complex due to new life-sustaining treatments. Researchers have therefore been attempting to develop computer-assisted medical diagnostic tools to aid physicians in this task.[1-3] This chapter describes a method for computer-based diagnosis that uses a probabilistic causal knowledge representation and a probabilistic inference technique.

Diagnosis is defined here as determining the most likely set of diseases to account for a set of case-specific patient findings. In probability terminology, the task is to find the diagnostic hypothesis H_j that maximizes the probability $P(H_j \mid F)$, where H_j is a set of one or more diseases and F is a set of findings. Thus in order to arrive at a diagnosis, it is necessary to determine the relative likelihood of different diagnostic hypotheses. This chapter focuses on the calculation of $P(H_j \mid F)$ for an arbitrary hypothesis H_j. Calculation of this probability for every H_j allows determination of the most likely diagnostic hypothesis. In large medical domains, this exhaustive approach may be too time-consuming. In such cases, more efficient hypothesis search techniques can be used.[4] Nonetheless, the latter search techniques also are based on the use of probabilities, which can be calculated using the methods discussed in this chapter.

Over the past 25 years, researchers in computer-assisted medical diagnosis have made extensive use of Bayes' formula[5-9] to calculate $P(H_j \mid F)$:

$$P(H_j \mid F) = \frac{P(F \mid H_j) \times P(H_j)}{P(F \mid H_j) \times P(H_j) + P(F \mid \text{not } H_j) \times P(\text{not } H_j)}$$

$$= \frac{P(F \mid H_j) \times P(H_j)}{\sum_{k=1}^{n} P(F \mid H_k) \times P(H_k)} \tag{1}$$

where $\mathbf{F}$ is a set of findings and $\mathbf{H}_j$ is a diagnostic hypothesis from among a set of n possible diagnostic hypotheses. Each hypothesis $\mathbf{H}_j$ consists of a set of diseases. The n diagnostic hypotheses constitute every possible subset of the diseases in the domain. Therefore within the domain, the n hypotheses are exhaustive and are mutually exclusive.

A computer diagnostic system based on Bayes' formula has the advantage of being a formal probabilistic system. In general, several benefits result from using a diagnostic method based on formal probability theory:

1. Probability as a field of mathematics is well developed. It aids researchers design computational methods for diagnosis, understand how these methods relate to previous research, and communicate them to other researchers.
2. Any assumptions made in the process of determining the likelihood of a hypothesis can be expressed unambiguously. It may help the user interpret the resulting score. It also may help the designer of the diagnostic algorithm to determine which assumptions to make when designing the program.
3. It is possible to use available statistical data *directly*.
4. It is possible to interface the hypothesis score (a probability) directly with other decision-making procedures, e.g., decision analysis programs.[10,11]

Thus using a formal probability-based system carries great attraction.

In addition, implementation of Bayes' formula yields formal systems that provide a means of using probabilities representing sensitivity information, i.e., $P(\text{findings} \mid \text{disease})$, and prevalence,* i.e., $P(\text{disease})$, rather than predictive value probabilities, i.e., $P(\text{disease} \mid \text{findings})$. The utility of the formula results from the greater availability of sensitivity and prevalence probabilities relative to predictive value probabilities. Conditional probabilities in medicine are largely available as sensitivities rather than as predictive value probabilities. Thus the literature is more likely to have data in the form of $P(\mathbf{F} \mid \mathbf{H}_j)$ than in the form of $P(\mathbf{H}_j \mid \mathbf{F})$. In addition, physicians often are more comfortable relating subjective estimates of $P(\mathbf{F} \mid \mathbf{H}_j)$ than they are those of $P(\mathbf{H}_j \mid \mathbf{F})$. In a like manner, $P(\mathbf{H}_j)$ usually either is available from known population statistics or can be estimated for a given population. Implementations of Bayes' formula, however, almost invariably make the following two assumptions:

1. *The conditional probabilities of findings given a diagnostic hypothesis are independent.* Thus $P(\mathbf{F} \mid \mathbf{H}_j)$, which is used in both the numerator and denominator of the last term in Eq. 1, is approximated by $P(f_1 \mid \mathbf{H}_j) \times \ldots \times P(f_m \mid \mathbf{H}_j)$, where $f_1, \ldots, f_m$ are the individual findings in the set $\mathbf{F}$.

---

*The term *prevalence* is used here to represent the probability of encountering a given disease or set of diseases within a given medical setting.

2. *A diagnostic hypothesis is a single disease from among a given set of diseases that are exhaustive and mutually exclusive.* That is, the patient's clinical condition corresponds to one and only one disease from among a given set of diseases.

Unfortunately, these assumptions are often invalid. Although in some domains the first assumption (conditional independence) may result in acceptable diagnostic accuracy,[9] there are domains in which the assumption is known to be invalid.[12,13] Therefore, we cannot rely on it to yield accurate diagnoses across all fields of medicine under all possible conditions.

The second assumption also is often invalid, particularly in complex cases in which multiple disease diagnoses are likely. It is for just these complex situations that a physician is most likely to seek a consultation.

In summary, most computer diagnostic programs that implement Bayes' formula have the advantages of being based on formal probability theory and of using more readily available statistics. However, in implementing Bayes' formula, they make assumptions that are often invalid.

We discuss a method herein that uses causal knowledge to represent the relations among diseases and findings in order to express the known probabilistic dependencies among them. This approach avoids the uniform assumption that findings are conditionally independent given diseases. Also, when calculating $P(\mathbf{H}_j \mid \mathbf{F})$ for a given diagnostic hypothesis $\mathbf{H}_j$, the method does not assume that $\mathbf{H}_j$ is a single disease. We emphasize here representation and inference concepts for probabilistic medical diagnosis, rather than computational efficiency issues.

Knowledge Representation

The graphical representation of probabilistic relations among events has been the subject of considerable research. *Markov models* form one such class of probabilistic graphical representations.[14,15] In the field of artificial intelligence, numerous systems have used a *directed graph* to represent probabilistic relations among events.[16,17] Often such graphs represent causal relations. A particular type of probabilistic graphical representation, called a *belief network,* has been independently defined and explored by several researchers. Belief networks[18] have also been termed *causal nets,*[19,20] *probabilistic cause–effect models,*[21] *probabilistic causal networks,*[4] and *influence diagrams.** [22,23]

---

*A belief network is a specialization of an influence diagram. An influence diagram represents decision alternatives and outcome values in addition to the probabilities of a belief network. The term *decision network* is perhaps a more intuitive name for an influence diagram, but it is not the standard term presently being used.

A primary advantage of a graphical representation of probabilistic relations is the efficiency that results in knowledge acquisition. It is necessary to consider only the known dependencies among variables (events) in a domain, rather than to assume that all variables are dependent on all other variables.[4,24] This approach generally leads to improved efficiency in the acquisition and representation of domain knowledge.

A belief network is one such graphical representation of probabilistic relations. It is a directed, acyclic graph in which nodes represent domain variables. For simplicity, we assume that the nodes represent propositional variables with a value of either true (T) or false (F). Probabilities are attached to nodes and to arcs or local groups of arcs. Figure 7.1 contains a simple belief network from the domain of medicine.† As shown in this figure, the graph is augmented by a set of probabilities. For example, the probability of a patient having a *brain tumor* (i.e., C = T) given that he has *metastatic cancer* (i.e., A = T) is 20%.‡ Belief network semantics require that *increased total serum calcium* and *brain tumor* be conditionally independent given *metastatic cancer*. If it were not so, further dependencies among the events would need to be represented by a more complex belief network. In the example, *coma* is caused by both *increased total serum calcium* and *brain tumor*. When an event is caused by multiple events, the probability of each effect given each combination of the causes must be represented. Generally, it is done explicitly with a table. For example, on the right of Figure 7.1 there is a table that specifies the probability of *D* = T for each possible state of the immediate predecessors of *D*. Although probability tables are often used for expressing probabilistic relations among events, analytic functional probabilistic relations can also be expressed between causes and effects.

Belief networks are capable of representing any joint probability space, such that any particular probability in that space can be computed from the explicitly represented probabilities. The key feature of belief networks is their explicit representation of conditional independence among events. We now formally define the conditional independence that is expressed in the structure of a belief network.[25,26] We need the following auxiliary definitions:

1. U is the set of all nodes in a given belief network.
2. A node x_j is a *direct predecessor* of node x_i if there is an arc from x_j to x_i.

---

†This medical example has been greatly simplified for the purpose of illustration; it is not intended to convey a realistic representation of all the probabilistic causal relations among the events shown.

‡Some probabilities are not shown in Figure 7.1 but they can be readily generated from the set of given probabilities. For example, $P(C = F \mid A = T) = 1 - P(C = T \mid A = T) = 1 - 0.2 = 80\%$.

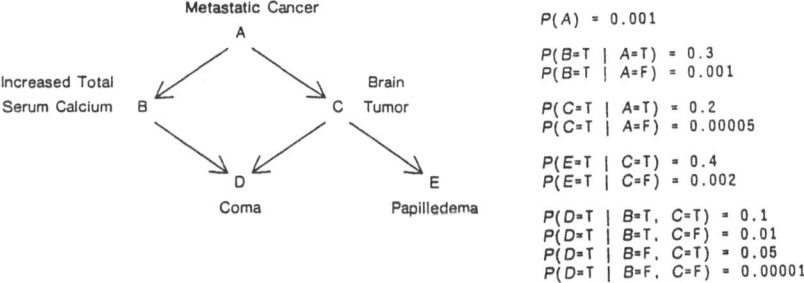

Metastatic Cancer
A

Increased Total
Serum Calcium   B   C   Brain
                                         Tumor

                D   E
              Coma   Papilledema

P(A) = 0.001

P(B=T | A=T) = 0.3
P(B=T | A=F) = 0.001

P(C=T | A=T) = 0.2
P(C=T | A=F) = 0.00005

P(E=T | C=T) = 0.4
P(E=T | C=F) = 0.002

P(D=T | B=T, C=T) = 0.1
P(D=T | B=T, C=F) = 0.01
P(D=T | B=F, C=T) = 0.05
P(D=T | B=F, C=F) = 0.00001

Figure 7-1. Example of a belief network.

3. $\mathbf{P}_i$ is the set of all direct predecessors of x_i.
4. A node x_k is a *successor* of node x_i if there is a directed path from x_i to x_k.
5. $\mathbf{S}_i$ is the set of all successors of x_i.
6. $\mathbf{S}_i'$ is the complement of the set of all successors of x_i, excluding node x_i itself. Thus $\mathbf{S}_i' = \mathbf{U} - \mathbf{S}_i - \{x_i\}$.
7. $\mathbf{Q}_i$ is the set of all possible subsets of $\mathbf{S}_i'$. In other words, $\mathbf{Q}_i$ is the power set of $\mathbf{S}_i'$.

For example, in the belief network in Figure 7-1, suppose that $x_i = D$. In this case, $\mathbf{U} = \{A, B, C, D, E\}$, $\mathbf{P}_i = \{B, C\}$, $\mathbf{S}_i = \emptyset$, $\mathbf{S}_i' = \{A, B, C, E\}$, and $\mathbf{Q}_i = \{\{\}, \{A\}, \{B\}, \{C\}, \{E\}, \{A, B\}, \{A, C\}, \{A, E\}, \{B, C\}, \{B, E\}, \{C, E\}, \{A, B, C\}, \{A, B, E\}, \{A, C, E\}, \{B, C, E\}, \{A, B, C, E\}\}$.
In general, for a given node x_i, a belief network containing x_i expresses the following conditional independence relation:

$$\text{For all sets } q \text{ in } \mathbf{Q}_i: P(\mathrm{x_i} \mid \mathbf{P}_i \cup q) = P(x_i \mid \mathbf{P}_i) \qquad (2)$$

This relation states that if the values of the direct predecessors of x_i are known with certainty, the probability of each value of x_i is independent of the value of other nodes that are not successors of x_i. In the previous example, knowing the values of nodes B and C is sufficient to determine the probability that node $D = T$, regardless of the values of nodes A and E. The absence of an arc from node A to node D is a statement that the probability distribution on the values of node D is conditionally independent of the value of node A, given the values of nodes B and C. In general, the absence of an arc from a node x_j in $\mathbf{S}_i'$ to node x_i indicates that x_i is conditionally independent of x_j, given the values of the nodes in $\mathbf{P}_i$.

Assume the n nodes in a given belief network have been labeled as x_1, $x_2, \ldots, x_n$, so that for each x_i there exists at least one member of $\mathbf{Q}_i$—call it q_i—such that $\{x_1, x_2, \ldots, x_{i-1}\} = \mathbf{P}_i \cup q_i$. Although we do not prove it here, such an ordering is always possible. The joint probability of some particular instantiation* of all n variables in a belief network therefore can be calculated as follows:

$$P(X_1, \ldots, X_n) = \prod_{i=1}^{n} P(X_i \mid X_1, \ldots, X_{i-1}) \tag{3}$$

$$\prod_{i=1}^{n} P(X_i \mid X_1, \ldots, X_{i-1}) = \prod_{i=1}^{n} P(X_i \mid \mathbf{P}_i \cup \mathbf{q}_i) \tag{4}$$

$$\prod_{i=1}^{n} P(X_i \mid \mathbf{P}_i \cup \mathbf{q}_i) = \prod_{i=1}^{n} P(X_i \mid \mathbf{P}_i) \tag{5}$$

The notation $X_1, \ldots, X_{i-1}$ is used as shorthand to specify the set of all X_j for $1 \le j < i$. Equation 3 follows from the definition of conditional probability. Equation 4 follows from the ordering condition on the x_i. Equation 5 follows from the conditional independence property of belief networks as expressed in Eq. 2. For example, consider the following calculation of the joint probability of all the variables in Figure 7-1 with values instantiated to true (T):

$$P(A = T, B = T, C = T, D = T, E = T) = \tag{6}$$
$$P (E = T \mid A = T, B = T, C = T, D = T) \times P(D = T, \mid$$
$$\qquad A = T, B = T, C = T) \times$$
$$\qquad P(C = T \mid A = T, B = T) \times P (B = T \mid A = T) \times P(A = T)$$

$$P(E = T \mid A = T, B = T, C = T, D = T) \times P(D = T \mid$$
$$\qquad A = T, B = T, C = T) \times \tag{7}$$
$$\qquad P(C = T \mid A = T, B = T) \times P(B = T \mid A = T) \times$$
$$\qquad P(A = T) =$$
$$P(E = T \mid C = T) \times P(D = T \mid B = T, C = T) \times P(C = T \mid$$
$$\qquad A = T) \times P(B = T \mid A = T) \times P(A = T) =$$
$$0.4 \times 0.1 \times 0.2 \times 0.3 \times 0.001 = 2.4 \times 10^{-6}$$

Equation 6 follows from Eq. 3; Eq. 7 follows from Eqs. 4 and 5. The complete joint probability space can be recovered from the belief network representation by calculating the joint probabilities that result from every possible instantiation of the n variables in the network. However, instead of representing all 2^n probabilities in the joint space, it is necessary to represent only $P(x_i \mid \mathbf{P}_i)$ for each node x_i in the network; this representation may require a total of many fewer than 2^n probabilities. For example, in Figure 7.1 only 11 probabilities are needed to represent the five-node belief network, rather than $2^5 - 1 = 31$.

Although an arc from x to y often is used to express that x causes y,

---

*The term *instantiated variable* is used to denote a variable with a known, assigned value. For example, an instantiated propositional variable would have an assigned value of either true (T) or false (F).

it need not be the interpretation of arcs in belief networks. For example, y may be only correlated with x, but not caused by x. Thus although belief networks are able to represent causal relations, they are not restricted to such causal interpretations. Although we continue to use a causal interpretation of belief networks in this chapter, it is important to realize that belief networks also can be used to represent noncausal rule-based systems that reason with uncertainty.

In summary, belief networks allow an explicit graphic representation of probabilistic conditional dependence and independence. This representation generally reduces the number of probability assessments needed (relative to the full joint probability space), and it sometimes reduces the computational complexity of probabilistic inference.

Probabilistic Inference

A diagnostic hypothesis (H_j) is an instantiated set of disease variables; an example is the set $H_1 = \{metastatic\ cancer = T\}$. The findings F are an instantiated set of finding variables; an example is the set $F_1 = \{increased\ total\ serum\ calcium = T, coma = F, papilledema = T\}$. Probabilistic inference is defined as the task of using a given belief network to calculate $P(H_j \mid F)$. The following formulas perform this calculation:

$$P(y_1, y_2, \ldots, y_n) = \prod_{i=1}^{n} P(y_i \mid P_i) \tag{8}$$

where y_i is equal to X_i (i.e., the instantiated value of variable x_i) if X_i is an instantiated variable in either H_j or F. Otherwise, y_i is equal to the uninstantiated variable x_i.

Equation 8 follows from Eqs. 3, 4, and 5.

$$P(H_j, F) = \sum_{y_i \notin (H_j \cup F)} P(y_1, y_2, \ldots, y_n) \tag{9}$$

Equation 9 sums the elements of the joint probability space that contain the instantiated variables in the hypothesis set H_j and in the finding set F. In effect, it "sums out" all the variables that are not instantiated variables in H_j and F.

$$P(z_1, z_2, \ldots, z_n) = \prod_{i=1}^{n} P(z_i \mid P_i) \tag{10}$$

where z_i is equal to X_i (i.e., the instantiated value of variable x_i) if X_i is an instantiated variable in F. Otherwise, z_i is equal to the uninstantiated variable x_i.

Equation 10 follows from Eqs. 3, 4, and 5.

$$P(F) = \sum_{z_i \notin F} P(z_1, z_2, \ldots, z_n) \tag{11}$$

Equation 11 sums the elements of the joint probability space that contain the instantiated variables in the finding set **F**. In effect, it "sums out" all the variables that are not instantiated variables in **F**.

$$P(\mathbf{H}_j \mid \mathbf{F}) = \frac{P(\mathbf{H}_j, \mathbf{F})}{P(\mathbf{F})} \qquad (12)$$

Equation 12 follows from the definition of conditional probability and is computed using Eqs. 9 and 11.

Example of Probabilistic Inference Using a Belief Network

Consider the calculation of the goal probability $P(metastatic\ cancer = \mathrm{T} \mid increased\ total\ serum\ calcium = \mathrm{T},\ coma = \mathrm{F},\ papilledema = \mathrm{T})$ using the belief network in Figure 7-1. To simplify the notation, we express it as $P(A = \mathrm{T} \mid B = \mathrm{T}, D = \mathrm{F}, E = \mathrm{T})$. Here $\mathbf{H}_j = \{A = \mathrm{T}\}$ and $\mathbf{F} = \{B = \mathrm{T}, D = \mathrm{F}, E = \mathrm{T}\}$. Using Eq. 12, the goal probability can be expressed as

$$
\begin{aligned}
&P(A = \mathrm{T} \mid B = \mathrm{T}, D = \mathrm{F}, E = \mathrm{T}) \\
&\qquad = \frac{P(A = \mathrm{T}, B = \mathrm{T}, D = \mathrm{F}, E = \mathrm{T})}{P(B = \mathrm{T}, D = \mathrm{F}, E = \mathrm{T})}
\end{aligned}
\qquad (13)
$$

The numerator of Eq. 13 is calculated as follows, using the sum-of-products operation in Eqs. 8 and 9:

$$
\begin{aligned}
&P(A = \mathrm{T}, B = \mathrm{T}, D = \mathrm{F}, E = \mathrm{T}) = P(A = \mathrm{T}, B = \mathrm{T}, C = \mathrm{F}, \\
&\quad D = \mathrm{F}, E = \mathrm{T}) + P(A = \mathrm{T}, B = \mathrm{T}, C = \mathrm{T}, D = \mathrm{F}, \\
&\quad E = \mathrm{T}) =
\end{aligned}
\qquad (14)
$$

$P(E = \mathrm{T} \mid C = \mathrm{F}) \times P(D = \mathrm{F} \mid B = \mathrm{T}, C = \mathrm{F}) \times P(C = \mathrm{F} \mid$
$\quad A = \mathrm{T}) \times P(B = \mathrm{T} \mid A = \mathrm{T}) \times P(A = \mathrm{T}) +$

$P(E = \mathrm{T} \mid C = \mathrm{T}) \times P(D = \mathrm{F} \mid B = \mathrm{T}, C = \mathrm{T}) \times P(C = \mathrm{T} \mid$
$\quad A = \mathrm{T}) \times P(B = \mathrm{T} \mid A = \mathrm{T}) \times P(A = \mathrm{T}) =$

$0.002 \times 0.99 \times 0.8 \times 0.3 \times 0.001 +$
$0.4 \times 0.9 \times 0.2 \times 0.3 \times 0.001 =$
$4.75 \times 10^{-7} + 2.16 \times 10^{-5} = 2.2 \times 10^{-5}$

Equation 14 sums the elements of the joint probability space that contain both the instantiated variables in the hypothesis set $\mathbf{H}_j$ and those in the finding set **F**. In this simple example the only variable that is not a member of $\mathbf{H}_j$ or **F** is C. Thus the right side of Eq. 14 is a summation over all values of variable C. Because C is a propositional variable (i.e., it has the value either T or F), it leads to the two terms shown in the sum. Equation 14 sums out the variable C, by summing over both values of C.

The denominator of Eq. 13 is calculated as follows, using the sum-of-products operation in Eqs. 10 and 11:

$P(B = T, D = F, E = T) =$

$\quad P(A = T, B = T, C = F, D = F, E = T) +$ (15)

$P(A = T, B = T, C = T, D = F, E = T) +$

$P(A = F, B = T, C = F, D = F, E = T) +$

$P(A = F, B = T, C = T, D = F, E = T) =$

$P(E = T \mid C = F) P(D = F \mid B = T, C = F) P(C = F \mid$
$\quad A = T) P(B = T \mid A = T) P(A = T) +$

$P(E = T \mid C = T) P(D = F \mid B = T, C = T) P(C = T \mid$
$\quad A = T) P(B = T \mid A = T) P(A = T) +$

$P(E = T \mid C = F) P(D = F \mid B = T, C = F) P(C = F \mid$
$\quad A = F) P(B = T \mid A = F) P(A = F) +$

$P(E = T \mid C = T) P(D = F \mid B = T, C = T) P(C = T \mid$
$\quad A = F) P(B = T \mid A = F) P(A = F) =$

$0.002 \times 0.99 \times 0.8 \times 0.3 \times 0.001 +$

$0.4 \times 0.9 \times 0.2 \times 0.3 \times 0.001 +$

$0.002 \times 0.99 \times 0.99995 \times 0.001 \times 0.999 +$

$0.4 \times 0.9 \times 0.00005 \times 0.001 \times 0.999 =$

$4.75 \times 10^{-7} + 2.16 \times 10^{-5} + 1.98 \times 10^{-6} + 1.80 \times 10^{-8} =$
$\quad 2.4 \times 10^{-5}$

Equation 15 sums the elements of the joint probability space that contain the instantiated variables in the finding set **F**. In the example, variables A and C are not members of set **F**. Thus the right side of Eq. 15 is a summation over all values of variables A and C, leading to the four terms shown. Combining Eqs. 14 and 15 leads to the following final result:

$$P(A = T \mid B = T, D = F, E = T) =$$
$$2.2 \times 10^{-5} / 2.4 \times 10^{-5} = 0.92$$

Probability Bounds

The probability of an event can be expressed as an interval rather than as a unique point value.[27-30] In particular, it is possible to place an upper and lower bound on any probability in a belief network.[4] For example, $P(B = T \mid A = T)$ might be bounded as $0.2 \leq P(B = T \mid A = T) \leq 0.4$, rather than being given a point probability of 0.3, as in Figure 7.1. A bounded probability expresses the belief that the probability value for an event lies in a specified interval, without making any commitment to where it lies within that interval. A bounded probability representation may be useful in the acquisition of subjective probabilities from an expert during the construction of a belief network. It does not force the expert to commit to a unique-valued probability when the expert has little confidence in such a point probability. A point probability can be expressed, when desired, by setting the upper and lower bound at the same value.

Probabilistic inference using bounded probabilities is a straightforward extension of the unique-valued probability calculations discussed above. In particular, $P(\mathbf{H}_j \mid \mathbf{F})$ in Eq. 12 is calculated twice instead of once. An upper bound on $P(\mathbf{H}_j \mid \mathbf{F})$ is calculated with Eq. 12 by calculating and using the maximum value of each term $P(y_1, y_2, \ldots, y_n)$ in Eq. 9, the maximum value of each term $P(z_1, z_2, \ldots, z_n)$ in Eq. 11 that is equal to a term in Eq. 9, and the minimum value of the remaining terms in Eq. 11. A lower bound on $P(\mathbf{H}_j \mid \mathbf{F})$ is calculated in an analogous manner. In effect, this method is a type of sensitivity analysis over all the probabilities in the belief network.

Representing probabilities with bounds sometimes results in inferred probabilities with very wide bounds, which in turn may lead to diagnostic hypotheses with probabilities that overlap. Consider the two diagnostic hypotheses $\mathbf{H}_1$ and $\mathbf{H}_2$, and a set of findings $\mathbf{F}$. Suppose that the bounds on $P(\mathbf{H}_1 \mid \mathbf{F})$ overlap those of $P(\mathbf{H}_2 \mid \mathbf{F})$. In this case, without additional knowledge, it is not possible to determine which hypothesis is the most probable. Thus, in general, bounding probabilities leads to a partial order on diagnostic hypotheses rather than to a total order. However, this partial order can be incrementally transformed into a total order by tightening the bounds on the probabilities in the belief network. This process might be guided by a program module that indicates those probability bounds in the belief network to which the bounds on $P(\mathbf{H}_j \mid \mathbf{F})$ are most sensitive. Often it is sufficient to merely establish a total order between a diagnostic hypothesis $\mathbf{H}_{\text{top}}$ and all other diagnostic hypotheses, where the lower bound of $\mathbf{H}_{\text{top}}$ is higher than the upper bound of any other hypothesis. A total order between $\mathbf{H}_{\text{top}}$ and all other diagnostic hypotheses can sometimes be established by obtaining additional findings about the patient. These additional findings may establish a total order by decreasing the overlap of bounds of diagnostic hypotheses. Thus tightening bounds among the belief network probabilities and obtaining additional findings are two possible methods for generating nonoverlapping bounds among diagnostic hypotheses to determine $\mathbf{H}_{\text{top}}$.

Computational Time Complexity

The algorithm discussed under Probabilistic Inference, above, is based on calculating Eq. 12 using Eqs. 8 through 11. Thus the computational complexity of this algorithm is equal to the computational complexity of calculating Eq. 12. Suppose there are n variables in a given belief network. The numerator of Eq. 12, which is computed using Eq. 9, requires summing over $n - \mid \mathbf{H}_j \cup \mathbf{F} \mid$ variables. If these variables are binary, this calculation requires $2^{n - \mid \mathbf{H}_j \cup \mathbf{F} \mid}$ summation steps. Each summation step requires a product of n probability terms, which is computed using Eq. 8. Thus the computational complexity of calculating the numerator of Eq. 12 is $n \, 2^{n \, - \, |H_j \cup F|}$. The denominator of Eq. 12 requires summing over $n - |F|$ variables. Thus its computational time complexity is $n \, 2^{n \, - \, |F|}$. The total computational complexity of probabilistic inference using this technique is the sum of the computational complexity of calculating the numerator and denominator of Eq. 12, which is equal to $n \, (2^{n \, - \, |H_j \cup F|} + 2^{n \, - \, |F|})$.

However, the summation in Eq. 9 is contained as a partial sum of Eq. 11. Thus by avoiding redundant calculations it is necessary to compute only the sum in Eq. 11, which leads to a total computational complexity of $n \, 2^{n \, - \, |F|}$.

This analysis indicates that the computation time increases rapidly as the number of nodes in the belief network increases. For example, to calculate the probability of a diagnostic hypothesis given 10 findings, a network of only 30 nodes requires $30 \times 2^{30 \, - \, 10} \approx 3 \times 10^7$ computation steps. Thus the probability inference algorithm discussed under Probabilistic Inference is impractical for belief networks that contain more than about 30 nodes. However, this algorithm is conceptually useful for understanding the fundamental operations that are necessary for probabilistic inference using belief networks.

A simple modification of that algorithm renders it much more efficient in many cases. Equations 8 through 11 perform calculations using *all* the variables in a given belief network. We represent these variables with the set U. The modified algorithm considers only a subset of U, which we call V. The set V consists of all the variables in U that are either in H_j or F, or that have successors that are in H_j or F. The products and sums in Eqs. 8 through 11 need only be taken over the variables in set V. Because V is often much smaller than U, this modified algorithm is typically much more efficient than the brute-force algorithm discussed above.

Other techniques have been developed for performing efficient probabilistic inference. These techniques typically deal with special classes of belief networks. For example, tree-structured networks containing n binary nodes with bounded branching can be calculated using on the order of n, e.g., $O(n)$, computational steps.[4] More generally, linear time algorithms have been developed for probabilistic inference using singly connected belief networks.*[18] However, in the worst cases, for inference using multiply connected networks, all current algorithms require an exponential number of computation steps as a function of the number of nodes in the belief network. In fact, this task is known to be NP-hard.[31] Thus it is

---

*A *singly connected belief network* contains at most one pathway (in the undirected sense) between any two nodes in the network. A *multiply connected belief network* contains at least two nodes that have more than one pathway between them. For example, the belief network in Figure 7.1 is multiply connected; removal of node A, B, C, or D would render it singly connected.

unlikely that any algorithm can be developed that can in the worst cases efficiently perform *exact* probabilistic inference. Here *exact probabilistic inference* is defined as probabilistic inference that produces a completely accurate, precise probability in the context of a given belief network. Therefore current research is focusing on solving special cases efficiently, finding efficient bounding algorithms, developing good heuristic algorithms, and determining if the worst cases arise often enough, or are complex enough, to make them of any practical concern in numerous medical domains. The formal framework of belief networks provides a well defined and coherent base from which to explore these various approaches to pragmatic reasoning under uncertainty in medicine.

Summary

Probabilistic inference using belief networks provides a coherent and axiomatically well defined method for building medical diagnostic systems. A belief network representation allows the efficient specification of a formal probabilistic medical knowledge base. The knowledge base can be a causal network, a rule base, or a combination of the two. The probabilities in the belief network can be bounded, rather than being specified as unique point values. This representation can then be used to determine the probability bounds of a diagnostic hypothesis given a set of findings. The calculation forms the foundation for a medical diagnostic system. However, exact probabilistic inference using belief networks can be computationally expensive.

This chapter described a brute-force approach to probabilistic inference that quickly becomes intractable as the size of the belief network increases. Nonetheless, this approach is conceptually instructive. Efficient techniques have been developed for probabilistic inference using special types of belief networks. However, probabilistic inference using belief networks remains computationally expensive in some complex cases. Current research is determining the cases that are of practical concern. Work is also focusing on finding acceptable, although inexact, solutions to even the theoretically most complex cases.

Acknowledgments. I wish to thank David Heckerman for valuable comments on this chapter. This work has been supported by grant LM-07033 from the National Library of Medicine. Computer facilities were provided by the SUMEX-AIM resource under NIH grant RR-00785.

References

1. Szolovits P (ed): Artificial Intelligence in Medicine. Boulder, CO: Westview Press, 1982.

2. Clancey WJ, Shortliffe EH (eds): Readings in Medical Artificial Intelligence: The First Decade. Reading, MA: Addison Wesley, 1984.
3. Reggia JA, Tuhrim S (eds): Computer-Assisted Medical Decision Making. New York: Springer-Verlag, 1985.
4. Cooper GF: NESTOR: A Computer-Based Medical Diagnostic Aid that Integrates Causal and Probabilistic Knowledge. PhD dissertation, Medical Information Sciences, Stanford University, 1984. CS report STAN-CS-84-1031.
5. Miller MC III, Westphal MC, Reigart JR, Barner C: Medical Diagnostic Models: A Bibliography. Ann Arbor, MI: University Microfilms International, 1977.
6. Warner HR, Toronto AF, Veasy LG, Stephenson R: A mathematical approach to medical diagnosis: application to congenital heart disease. JAMA 177: 177, 1961.
7. Wagner G, Tauta P, Wolber U: Problems of medical diagnosis—a bibliography. Methods Inf Med 17: 55, 1978.
8. Leaper DJ, Horrocks JC, Staniland JR, deDombal FT: Computer-assisted diagnosis of abdominal pain using estimates provided by clinicians. Br Med J 4: 350, 1972.
9. DeDombal FT, Leaper DJ, Horrocks JC, Staniland JR, McCain AP: Human and computer-aided diagnosis of abdominal pain: further report with emphasis on performance. Br Med J 1: 376, 1974.
10. Schwartz WB, Gorry GA, Kassirer JP, Essig A: Decision analysis and clinical judgement. Am J Med 55: 459, 1973.
11. Weinstein MC, Fineberg HV, Elstein AS, Frazier HS, Neuhauser D, Neutra RR, McNeil BJ: Clinical Decision Analysis. Philadelphia: Saunders, 1980.
12. Norusis MJ, Jacquez JA: Diagnosis. I. Symptom nonindependence in mathematical models for diagnosis. Comput Biomed Res 8: 156, 1975.
13. Fryback DG: Bayes' theorem and conditional nonindependence of data in medical diagnosis. Comput Biomed Res 11: 423, 1978.
14. Kemeny JG, Snell JL, Knapp AW: Denumerable Markov Chains. New York: Springer Verlag, 1976.
15. Darroch JN, Lauritzen SL, Speed TP: Markov fields and log-linear interaction models for contingency tables. Ann Statist 8: 522, 1980.
16. Duda RO, Hart PE, Nilsson NJ: Subjective Bayesian methods for rule-based inference systems. p. 1075. In: Proceedings of the 1976 National Computer Conference. New York: AFIPS Press, 1976.
17. Weiss JM, Kulikowski CA, Amarel S, Safir A: A model-based method for computer-aided medical decision-making. Artif Intell 11: 145, 1978.
18. Pearl J: Fusion, propagation, and structuring in belief networks. Artif Intell 29: 241, 1986.
19. Good IJ: A causal calculus (I). Br J Philos Sci 11: 305, 1961.
20. Good IJ: A causal calculus (II). Br J Philos Sci 12: 43, 1961.
21. Rousseau WF: A method for computing probabilities in complex situations. Technical report 6252-2. Stanford, CA: Stanford University Center for Systems Research, 1968.
22. Howard RA, Matheson JE: Readings on the Principles and Applications of Decision Analysis. 2nd Ed. Menlo Park, CA: Strategic Decisions Group, 1984.
23. Shachter RD: Evaluating influence diagrams. Operations Res 34: 871, 1986.

24. Pearl J, Verma TS: The logic of representing dependencies by directed graphs. In: Proceedings of the AAAI. Seattle: American Association for Artificial Intelligence, 1987.

25. Shachter RD: Intelligent probabilistic inference. p. 371. In Kanal LN, Lemmer JF (eds): Uncertainty in Artificial Intelligence. Amsterdam: North Holland, 1986.

26. Heckerman DE, Horvitz EJ: On the expressiveness of rule-based systems for reasoning under uncertainty. In: Proceedings of the AAAI. Seattle: American Association for Artificial Intelligence, 1987.

27. Keynes JM: A Treatise on Probability. London: Macmillan, 1921.

28. Koopman BO: The axioms and algebra of intuitive probability. Ann Mathematics 41: 269, 1940.

29. Good IJ: Subjective probability as the measure of a non-measureable set. p. 319. In: Logic, Methodology, and Philosophy of Science: Proceedings of the 1960 International Congress. Stanford, CA: Stanford University Press, 1962. Also in: Good Thinking: The Foundations of Probability and Its Applications. Minneapolis: University of Minnesota Press, 1983.

30. Kyburg HE Jr: Bayesian and non-Bayesian evidential updating. Artif Intell 31: 271, 1987.

31. Cooper GF: Probabilistic inference using belief networks is NP-hard. Technical report KSL-87-27. Stanford, CA: Medical Computer Science Group, Knowledge Systems Laboratory, Stanford University, 1987.

8
Using Causal Knowledge to Create Simulated Patient Cases: CPCS Project as an Extension of INTERNIST-1

Ronnie C. Parker and Randolph A. Miller

Expert systems for medical diagnosis require associated knowledge bases. A dichotomy, based on depth of causal representation, has been made by various researchers between the types of medical expert system knowledge bases. "Shallow" knowledge bases, such as that of the INTERNIST-1 program,[1] do not contain detailed representations of causality (i.e., they do not represent mechanisms by which a disease process causes clinical abnormalities in a given patient), whereas "deep," or "second-generation" expert systems, such as the ABEL program developed by Patil et al.,[2] contain sufficient causal information to make qualitative and quantitative predictions about pathophysiologic abnormalities in a given patient case.

During the mid-1970s an attempt was made by one of the authors to use the INTERNIST-1 knowledge base to create artificial "synthetic" patient cases for educational use by medical students. It was found that the "shallowness" of the INTERNIST-1 knowledge base prevented the successful generation of realistic patient cases. During the early 1980s a new format for knowledge representation was developed that corrected some of the known deficiencies of the INTERNIST-1 approach. The computer-based patient case simulation (CPCS) project made use of this new format for knowledge representation to successfully generate "simulated patients" de novo from the information contained in its expanded knowledge base. Yet the price of incorporating causality into the original format of the INTERNIST-1 knowledge base was substantial. The complexity of the experimental CPCS knowledge base was so great that it was impossible to maintain over long periods of time or to extend across the various specialties of internal medicine.

Two important concepts resulted from work on CPCS. First, a diagnostic program, even one that incorporates "deep" causal modeling, may contain undetected inadequacies in its knowledge base that can be uncovered only by attempting to run the diagnostic program "in reverse." The authors propose a "Turing test" for causal modeling in a diagnostic

From *Proceedings, 11th Symposium on Computer Applications in Medical Care*, pp. 473–480, © 1987, Institute of Electrical and Electronics Engineers, Inc. Reprinted with permission.

expert system: if a diagnostic program's knowledge base cannot be used to automatically construct artificial patient cases that cannot be distinguished by experts from an abstracted genuine patient case, there are deficiencies in that knowledge base. Whether such deficiencies are critical enough to influence the diagnostic behavior of the expert system is a separate issue. Second, and more important, is that developers of expert systems should take a balanced approach when deciding how "deep" to incorporate causal knowledge into any new expert system. "Deeper" is not always better. The functional requirements of a system should be taken into account when including causal knowledge to any arbitrary depth.

Case for Not Using Causal Modeling

There are reasons why the developers of an expert system might not include "deep" causal information in the expert system's knowledge base. The first reason is that causal modeling is in itself limited. As Blois[3] pointed out, medical theories and medical explanations are expressed at a higher level of conceptualization (interpretation and integration) than are theories and explanations in the physical sciences. For example, one does not often explain a patient's clinical abnormalities in terms of atomic bonding and subatomic forces.

A second factor limiting causal modeling in medical expert systems is that across all disciplines of medicine there is insufficient fundamental knowledge about the true cause of observed phenomena to allow detailed representation. Clinical medicine remains to a large extent an empiric science. Modern medicine cannot explain why penicillin causes urticaria in one patient and Stevens-Johnson syndrome in another, even though the mechanisms of the allergic reactions themselves are moderately well understood. In many disciplines, clinical observation is a more powerful methodology for defining a disease entity than is the development of a theoretical model of the disease. Our earliest characterizations of legionellosis, toxic shock syndrome, and acquired immunodeficiency syndrome (AIDS) were as clinical syndromes; only after subsequent years of research were the causative agents for the syndromes identified.

A third reason not to include causal models in expert systems is that a causal model may introduce undue complexity in a program's function. This "limiting" approach to causal reasoning has applicability to physicians as well as computer programs. Many cognitive theories of diagnosis assert that physicians "recognize" diseases by their patterns of presentation, just as an individual can recognize a friend's voice on the telephone without consciously invoking complex reasoning strategies. Currently, physicians are taught to think about diseases from a pathophysiologic perspective, but one could argue that it teaches only complicated mnemonics by which physicians are able to remember what can happen to patients with a given disease. Greek physicians were able to make clinical diagnoses of various disorders, even though their theories of the causes of the disorders, which invoked imbalances among the four basic elements, were probably incorrect. In the realm of expert systems, the "shallow" INTERNIST-1 program performs remarkably well for diagnosis in the broad field of internal medicine.[1] Although a certain number of cases presented to INTERNIST-1 cannot be solved because of the lack of causal reasoning by the system, the goal of constructing a deep causal knowledge base for the INTERNIST-1 program is unobtainable in practical terms. Fully 25 person-years have been devoted to building and maintaining the "shallow" knowledge base of INTERNIST-1, which is only about 80 percent complete. The authors estimate that building a "deep" causal knowledge base would be close to an order of magnitude more difficult, requiring several person-centuries of labor to complete—not a worthwhile undertaking given the current life-span of federal and private research grants and of individual academic careers.

INTERNIST-1/QMR Knowledge Base

INTERNIST-1 was developed during the early 1970s to solve complex diagnostic problems in internal medicine.[1,4] Continued development of this project is under way in the form of Quick Medical Reference (QMR), which uses similar, but extended structures in its knowledge representation.[5,6]

The knowledge represented in INTERNIST-1/QMR consists of 575 diseases in the field of internal medicine. The information about a given disease, referred to as its *disease profile,* is a linear undifferentiated list of all of the known clinical manifestations (historical patient findings, clinical symptoms, clinically demonstrable physical findings, and laboratory data) that have been found, through literature review, to occur in patients with the given disease. Associated with each of the clinical manifestations of a disease profile are two numbers, the *evoking strength* and the *frequency,* which represent the strength of the association of the manifestation to the disease in both directions. That is, the evoking strength is a number on a scale of 0 to 5 that answers the question, "If this finding is present in a patient, how strongly should the represented disease be considered as being present?" An evoking strength of 5 for a manifestation is considered to be pathognomonic. The frequency number is on a scale of 1 to 5 and answers the question, "If a patient has the represented disease, how often would the finding be present?" A frequency of 5 means that all of the patients with the disease have the finding.

In addition to this "flat" list of all of the known clinical manifestations comprising a disease profile, there are associations *(links)* from the represented disease to other represented diseases. These disease links detail the various types of relations between diseases (e.g., disease A causes disease B, disease A precedes disease B), and here too the linked diseases have associated evoking strength and frequency numbers representing the same strengths of association as for the findings. This combination of the clinical manifestations of a disease along with the disease's links represent what is called the disease profile. Table 8.1 is an abridged list of the information contained in the INTERNIST-1/QMR disease profile of *ascending cholangitis*. The leftmost column of numbers associated with each item is the evoking strength (0 to 5 scale) and the other column is the frequency (1 to 5 scale).

Causal information is represented in the existing INTERNIST-1/QMR knowledge base by the links among diseases. That is, there is a link from *diabetic ketoacidosis* to *diabetes mellitus* representing the fact that if a patient has diabetic ketoacidosis that knowledge is pathognomonic for the existence of the parent disease diabetes mellitus; and, conversely, diabetic ketoacidosis occurs in a few patients with diabetes mellitus. There are also direct causal links whenever a disease is reported verifiably to cause another disease. For example, the disease *Takayasu's arteritis* has been reported to cause *abdominal aortic aneurysm* only rarely; conversely, if a patient has *abdominal aortic aneurysm,* only rarely would *Takayasu's arteritis* be thought of as the cause. It is not widely appreciated that among the 575 "diseases" in the INTERNIST-1/QMR knowledge base some 85 to 90 pathophysiologic states, or clinical syndromes, have been represented as diseases. Examples of such syndromes include secondary aldosteronism, acute cardiogenic pulmonary congestion, nephrotic syndrome, various forms of ascites, chronic renal failure ("uremia"), and various forms of portal hypertension.

There are limitations of this form of knowledge representation, however.[1] The degree of severity of individual manifestations has not been well represented (e.g., *potassium serum decreased*), and the degree of severity of the individual diseases has not been represented. Pathophysiologic knowledge of the causes of manifestations within disease profiles has not been represented, and a disease profile contains an admixture of demographic and predisposing data as well as manifestations that are actually caused by the disease process. Anatomic reasoning is not described; and lastly, the representation of time is dealt with only crudely.

Computer-Based Patient Case Simulator

An interesting question regarding the INTERNIST-1 knowledge base arose during the mid-1970s: In what ways could the knowledge base be used for education as well as for diagnosis? One potential use that was envisioned was to construct "artificial patients" that would allow physicians

Table 8.1. Disease Profile of Ascending Cholangitis in the INTERNIST-1/QMR Format

0	2	AGE 26 to 55
0	3	AGE gtr than 55
2	4	BILE duct obstruction Hx
2	3	BILIARY tract surgery Hx
2	3	JAUNDICE intermittent Hx
0	3	SEX female
0	3	SEX male
1	3	URINE dark Hx
1	2	ABDOMEN pain acute
1	2	ABDOMEN pain colicky
1	2	ABDOMEN pain epigastrium
1	2	ABDOMEN pain epigastrium unrelieved by antacid
1	1	ABDOMEN pain exacerbation with breathing
1	1	ABDOMEN pain exacerbation with cough
1	2	ABDOMEN pain noncolicky
.		
.		
.		
3	5	LIVER biopsy periportal infiltration neutrophil <S>

Associated diagnoses for ascending cholangitis

CAUS-BY 3 4	stricture of bile duct
CAUS-BY 2 2	carcinoma of bile duct
CAUS-BY 2 2	carcinoma of head of pancreas
CAUS-BY 2 2	choledocholithiasis
CAUS 2 2	pyogenic liver abscess
CAUS-BY 1 2	carcinoma of gallbladder
PDIS-BY 1 2	hepatic artery aneurysm
CAUS-BY 1 2	sclerosing cholangitis
CAUS 1 1	amyloidosis systemic
PDIS-BY 1 1	congenital hepatic fibrosis
CAUS-BY 1 1	echinococcal cyst <S> of liver
PDIS 1 1	endocarditis acute infective left heart
PDIS 11	endocarditis infective right heart
COIN 1 1	hemobilia
CAUS 1 1	hepatic amyloidosis
CAUS 1 1	renal amyloidosis

in training to somehow "work up" patients and arrive at diagnoses in these "artificial patients" without incurring any risk of harm to actual patients. As a preliminary effort, the TEST program was developed. This program used the previously described format for disease information of INTERNIST-1/QMR. The TEST program would randomly choose one of the diseases in the knowledge base (remaining unknown to the user) and then randomize the order of that disease's list of manifestations. The program then went on to display three of these manifestations at a time, at which point the user was prompted to guess at the diagnosis from which those manifestations were taken. After entering the guessed diagnosis, a score was rendered that represented a crude estimate of the similarity of the two ("real" and "user's guessed") diagnosis. To the rudimentary TEST program, a feature was added that allowed the user to perform a crude sort of patient "work-up." Users could enter manifestations they thought might occur in their postulated disease and receive the information that indeed the manifestation did occur in the "real" diagnosis or that it did not. Additionally, a crude "cost" of requesting the manifestation was estimated, and this "cost" was factored into the score the user received. With the information gathered during the "work-up," the user would hopefully be better able to arrive at the "real" diagnosis that the machine was considering.

The TEST program had known deficiencies. The program did not simulate a patient, it merely presented manifestations that might occur in any patient with the selected disease, using the entire disease profile of the selected disease as a template from which to pick. For example, the manifestations list of *hepatitis acute viral* contains both *hepatomegaly present* and *liver small by percussion* as findings, and therefore both could be present in the TEST program's case presentation. Such contradictions would not occur in an actual patient. Another problem with the TEST program was that it did not create patient cases with the simultaneous occurrence of diseases that are interrelated by disease links in the IN-TERNIST-1/QMR knowledge base. For example, *micronodal cirrhosis, sinusoidal or postsinusoidal portal hypertension,* and *transudative ascites* are all listed separately within the INTERNIST-1/QMR knowledge base, and the TEST program was incapable of using that knowledge when presenting manifestations to the user. This situation would result in the manifestation of, for example, *hematemesis gross* always being absent when the machine was presenting a case of *Laennec's cirrhosis*.

In an effort to correct the deficiencies within the current representation scheme of INTERNIST-1/QMR, as well as to develop a knowledge base of sufficient caliber to simulate patients, a new knowledge base was constructed that used a new representation scheme. The Computer-based Patient Case Simulator (CPCS) project was started that incorporated the new format of knowledge representation.

CPCS Representation of Disease States

To overcome the deficiencies in the INTERNIST-1/QMR representation of knowledge, as well as in the TEST program, a new representation scheme was developed. A subset of liver diseases was chosen to be the domain for the new CPCS knowledge representation scheme.

Before disease redefinition was undertaken, the format for the manifestations (findings) had to be redesigned in order to better represent the interrelations of the findings themselves. In the INTERNIST-1/QMR knowledge base, a manifestation is a simple, nonparseable text string corresponding to an individual patient finding. Table 8.2 shows examples of INTERNIST-1/QMR manifestations dealing with abdominal pain. A medically knowledgeable individual is capable of understanding the interrelations of the findings, but these relations are only crudely represented in the INTERNIST-1/QMR knowledge base.[7] In the new format for manifestation definition, findings were defined with careful attention to what was being measured or described. The findings consisted in a frame structure that contained the following slots: finding name, status descriptor (the terminology associated with the finding in a patient case or disease profile), anatomic site descriptor, qualifier list (potentially modifying descriptors). This frame notation allowed more exact representation of the clinical manifestations of diseases as well as an explicit representation of what is "normal" and what is not.

Three categories of illnesses were allowed in the new CPCS knowledge base: diseases, facets, and subdivisions. Diseases represented the terminal endpoint of the diagnostic reasoning process and, for the most part, cor-

Table 8.2. INTERNIST-1/QMR Manifestations Dealing with Abdominal Pain

ABDOMEN pain acute
ABDOMEN pain chronic
ABDOMEN pain colicky
ABDOMEN pain epigastrium
ABDOMEN pain epigastrium recurrent attack or attacks Hx
ABDOMEN pain epigastrium relieved by antacid
ABDOMEN pain epigastrium relieved by food
ABDOMEN pain epigastrium seasonal Hx
.
.
.
ABDOMEN pain right upper quadrant exertional Hx
ABDOMEN pain right upper quadrant recurrent attack or attacks Hx
ABDOMEN pain severe
ABDOMEN pain suprapubic
CHEST pain substernal migrating to back or abdomen

responded to diseases as conceived in the INTERNIST-1/QMR knowledge base. Twelve diseases were identified in the domain of hepatobiliary diseases and functioned as the highest level of diagnostic resolution. Where applicable, each disease was described for three levels of severity: mild, moderate, and severe. Facets were the next category of described illness and represented intermediate pathophysiologic states or processes that made up diseases and thus were separately identifiable entities that represented a common pathway for the existence of a collection of manifestations. As such, one facet could be involved in potentially more than one disease. Subdivisions were the last category of illness in the CPCS knowledge base and represented subdivisions of either diseases or facets. There were two types of subdivision. The first type represented an organ system involvement by a disease process that could at times present as an illness itself. For example, patients with systemic lupus erythematosus can develop renal and central nervous system involvement; on some occasions, though, a patient may present with purely renal lupus or pure lupus cerebritis, with little or no signs of the systemic disease or of other organ system involvement. The second type of subdivision separated various mutually exclusive (either on an etiologic or a nosologic basis) forms of an illness. For example, the disease acute viral hepatitis in the new CPCS knowledge base was to have four subdivisions representing the unique features of hepatitis A, hepatitis B, delta hepatitis, and non-A non-B hepatitis.

This organization of the knowledge base allowed for inheritance of the manifestations of lower level items (subdivisions or facets) by the higher level diseases. This inheritance was not of a strict "isa" hierarchy though, as there is embedded probabilistic information in the knowledge base representing the encountered occurrence of the inherited item across all facets for a given disease, in addition to the probabilities listed under each facet.

With the new CPCS knowledge representation system, the definitions of these illnesses were divided into separate compartments, which helped clarify causal attribution. The compartments thus represented slots in a frame-based representation scheme with allowable fillers coming from instantiated manifestations (in the new frame-based structure also). The following separate slots for manifestations of disease existed:

Demographics: This slot contained information about the age, sex, and race distributions of the illness. Where it was possible, this information was subdivided for all of the represented severity forms of the illness.

General predisposing factors: This slot contained information about manifestations that, if one is present in a patient, place the patient at increased risk of developing the described illness. Also, there is information that describes how often at least one of these predisposing factors is present in patients presenting with the disease. It is assumed that, in any single patient, one such factor, at most, would be present.

Independent risk factors: This slot contained information about manifestations that, each of which, could place patients at risk of developing the described illness. These risk factors are distinct from the general predisposing factors in that if only one of the predisposing factors is present the other predisposing factors are not required or expected to be present. For the independent factors, each could make a contribution to the presence or absence of the disease. The manifestations in this and the preceding section, then, were findings that contributed to the illness but that were not specifically caused by the illness.

General effects: This slot contained information about the clinical manifestations observed in patients with the illness; furthermore, these manifestations are explained by more than one linked pathophysiologic state (facet) of the illness. The manifestations in this slot were those that result from multiple causes in patients with the illness. This slot allowed the assignment of an overall evoking strength and frequency for the manifestations that could be caused by different facets. For example, vomiting is observed in patients with some diseases because of potentially many causes; in those diseases this slot would contain the overall assessment of the relation of vomiting to that disease.

Specific effects: This slot contained information about the clinical manifestations observed in patients with the illness and also are recognized to be specifically caused by the illness, but not by mechanisms that are represented as facets. For example, anemia is known to cause skin pallor, so this type of information would be represented here.

Characteristic effects: This slot contained information about the clinical manifestations thought of as being even more strongly associated with an illness, i.e., present "by definition." For example, the hematocrit values of patients with anemia would be represented in this slot.

Academically known clinically contraindicated effects: This slot contained findings that we know (through research) are caused by the illness but that should not be used in routine clinical practice to determine if the illness is present in a patient. For example, we know that renal leptospirosis causes changes in the interstitial areas of the kidney on biopsy, but it would not be proper to do a renal biopsy on someone suspected of having renal leptospirosis to confirm the diagnosis.

Manifestations making diagnosis untenable: This slot contained those manifestations that would preclude the described illness as ever being present. For example, male sex precludes the diagnosis of toxemia of pregnancy, and a history of past cholecystectomy precludes a current diagnosis of acute cholecystitis.

Links: This slot contained information identifying relations between the illness being profiled and other components of the knowledge base (other diseases, facets, or subdivisions). For example, the information that acute fatty liver of pregnancy is a complication of pregnancy, can cause anemia, can cause gastritis, can cause hepatocellular inflammation, and can cause hepatomegaly would all be represented in this slot of the new knowledge base.

With this representation scheme, whenever a disease representation is "flushed out" to its clinical manifestations, it contains an admixture of findings that are directly attributable to the disease, as well as those findings that occur in the definition of subsumed facets and subdivisions.

A representative disease profile of *ascending cholangitis* in this knowledge representation scheme is shown in Table 8.3. Associated with each manifestation in the disease profile is a set of five numbers: The first two designate the traditional INTERNIST-1/QMR evoking strength and frequency, respectively; and the next three designate the frequency (0 to 5 scale) of the manifestation in the mild, moderate, and severe forms of the disease, respectively. This disease profile also demonstrates the use of the new format for finding representation. Several benefits were achieved with these changes in the CPCS representation format for the knowledge base. Qualifiers (modifiers) of patient findings were now more clearly associated with the findings being modified, and thus more appropriate differential diagnoses could theoretically be formed with the more precise patient case finding description. For example, it would be evident which pain was severe when multiple abdominal pains were described in a patient. Also, with the probabilistic information in the knowledge base, as well as the inheritance of lower level illness information by higher level illnesses, it became possible to attribute a finding in an artificially generated case to a more exact pathophysiologic entity than was possible in the INTERNIST-1/QMR representation. In the analysis of a case, it would be possible to assign the cause of an observed manifestation to several potential levels of defined illnesses, which allows better analysis of the case. Another of the major benefits was that the new disease, facet, and subdivision profiles contained findings and links that were relatively independent of each other because dependent findings share a common etiology, which then places them in a facet representing the common mechanism. Finally, by explicitly representing what is "normal" for findings, a more accurate case synthesis would be achieved than with the previous INTERNIST-1/QMR format.

CPCS Program Description

With the new CPCS format for knowledge representation, a computer program was written that would use this information to generate data representing a simulated patient. CPCS was written in the Franz LISP dialect of LISP, and the general method of case generation is summarized in the following statements:

1. A list of all of the allowable diagnoses is generated from which one is chosen to simulate a patient.

Table 8.3. Disease Profile of Ascending Cholangitis in the CPCS Format

Demographics
    Age (btw 16 25) (0 1 (1 1 1))
    Age (btw 26 55) (0 2 (2 2 2))
    Age (gtr than 55) (0 3 (3 3 3))
    Sex female (0 3 (3 3 3))
    Sex male (0 3 (3 3 3))

General predisposing factors
    General predisposing factor present true (0 4 (4 4 4))
    Bile duct obstruction history positive prior to present illness (2 4 (4 4 4))
    Surgery: history positive biliary tract surgery prior to present illness
    (2 2 (2 2 2))

Independent risk factors

General effects

Specific effects
    WBC total in thousands (btw 4 13.9) (0 3)
    WBC neutrophils percentage increased (0 4)
    Fever intermittent (1 5 (5 5 5))
    Gas in biliary tract present (3 2 (0 0 2))
    Neutrophilic cells infiltrating interlobular bile ducts present (3 5 (5 5 5))
    Periportal infiltration neutrophils (3 5 (5 5 5))
    WBC total in thousands (btw 14 30) (0 4 (4 4 4))
    WBC total in thousands (gtr than 30) (1 2 (0 1 2))

Characteristic findings

Academically known clinically contraindicated effects

Manifestations making diagnosis untenable

Links
    Source biliary colic
        Link type embodies facet
    Source cholestasis
        Link type embodies facet
    Source febrile response to microbial pyrogens
        Link type embodies facet
    Source hepatocellular inflammation and or necrosis
        Link type embodies facet
    Source hepatomegaly
        Link type complicated by facet
    Source peritoneal irritation right upper quadrant
        Link type embodies facet

2. A severity of the chosen disease is randomly picked using a weighting method based on the frequencies of the various severities.

3. All of the disorders (other diseases, subdivisions, and facets) that are linked in a causal manner (i.e., those disorders that can have as a cause the chosen disease) are reviewed and selected as "present" or "absent" in the simulated case. Based on the frequency of these linked conditions, the secondary disorders are then randomly designated as being present or not (again taking into account the frequency with which the chosen disease is caused by the linked disease).

4. A severity for each linked disorder (designated as present in the simulated case) is then assigned based on the frequencies of occurrence of the three severity forms of the linked disorder, in relation to the primary disease.

5. After generation of these first-order disease links the second-order disease links are generated using as the primary disease each of the first-order linked disorders. This step results in a combined list, to three levels of depth, of disorders designated as being present in the simulated case. The process of generating this list of disease entities makes extensive use of causal information that is contained within the knowledge base.

6. Using this list of disease processes that are present in the simulated patient, a list of the findings present in the simulated patient is generated. This process uses the knowledge base's causal information that associates a given clinical manifestation with a given disease entity (or facet or subdivision). Also used is the knowledge of the frequency of the possible finding in each severity of disease entity with which the finding is associated.

7. After generation of this list of the findings in the simulated patient, the computer presents a brief case description to the user. It consists in the patient's age, sex, and a few history, physical examination, or simple laboratory findings.

8. The user then proceeds to perform a "work-up" on the simulated patient by posing questions about specific manifestations that may or may not be present in the simulated case. If the manifestation is indeed present among the findings in the simulated patient, the program relays that information. If the manifestation was not present in the simulated case, a value for the finding within its "normal range" is generated. However, if the importance of the finding was low enough (so clinically its presence or absence does not add much information), the program occasionally gives a falsely positive answer (i.e., generates a "red herring"). If the manifestation were a laboratory test, the program would make up an appropriate numeric value to portray to the user. Once the user stops posing questions to the program, the program displays all of the findings and diseases that were considered to be active in the current simulated case. This display allows the user to receive feedback about actual manifestations that were present in the simulated patient as well as the diagnoses that were present.

Table 8.4 demonstrates an actual case being run. It shows the initial interaction with the user and then how the user would elucidate the set of findings in the simulated patient. As can be seen in the example case, the program, as it was developed, does a reasonable job of simulating the findings present in a patient with a given disease process. The use of the program does, however, require knowledge of the specific vocabulary in the knowledge base. Also, the final list of the findings and disease processes displayed to the user remains in its raw LISP form. The program demonstrated that it indeed was possible for a computer program to use a knowledge base (that had a considerable amount of causal knowledge) to generate consistent simulated patients. The algorithm involved with the case generation makes extensive use of causal information obtained in the linked illnesses (facets, subdivisions, and other "terminal level" diseases), as well as the information that pertains to the clinically observed manifestations being caused by a specific disease process (or facet or subdivision). This method ensures that, from the standpoint of observed clinical phenomenon, information portrayed to the user is consistent.

Table 8.4. Sample CPCS Run

The patient is a 34-year-old man. He presents with the following manifestations:
  Temperature 38.4°C
  Joint articular swelling and erythema, localized or diffuse
  Bilirubinuria

Enter finding or nil to stop: liver size
  (*Note:* at this point, the program would recapitulate all of the findings that are known about the patient. To save space, only the results of the asked-about finding are shown.)
Liver size normal

Enter finding or nil to stop: SGPT (blood)
  SGPT (blood) 199 mIU/ml

Enter finding or nil to stop: antigen-HBsAg
  Antigen-HBsAg positive

Enter finding or nil to stop: antinuclear antibody titer
  Antinuclear antibody titer normal

Enter finding or nil to stop: skin rash maculopapular
  Skin rash maculopapular absent, localized or diffuse

Enter finding or nil to stop: drug administration
  Drug administration true nitrofurantoin prior to present illness

Table 8.4. Continued

Enter finding or nil to stop: WBC eosinophil count
   WBC eosinophil count normal

Enter finding or nil to stop: fever variability with time
   Fever variability with time absent all categories

Enter finding or nil to stop: nil

Diagnosis: chronic active hepatitis severity 3
   (Demographics ((sex male) (age 34 years)))
   (General-predisposing-factors
      ((history
         (drug-administration true—nitrofurantoin prior to present-illness))))
   (Independent-risk-factors
      ((history
         (family-history positive; jaundice prior to present illness))
      (lab3 (HLA-type positive dw3))))
   (General effects
      ((symptom (appetite decreased))
      (observation
         (weight recent change in percent: 27%)
         (urine—gross inspection: abnormal ((Urine description dark-color)))
         (temperature 38.4°C)
         (skin: purpura or ecchymosis present, localized or diffuse)
         (jaundice present ((clinical time course acute))))
      (lab0 (SGOT blood 57 mIU/ml)
         (hemoglobin-blood 10.2 g/dl)
         (hematocrit-blood 31%)
         (cholesterol-blood decreased)
         (bilirubinuria present)
         (bilirubin-blood-total 5.7 mg/dl))
      (lab1 (urobilinogen-urine increased)
         (SGPT-blood 199 mIU/ml)
         (serum albumin decreased)
         (prothrombin time 1.6 times normal)
         (bilirubin-blood-conjugated increased))
      (lab4 (focal necrosis and inflammation of hepatocytes present))))
   (Specific effects
      ((observation
         (joint-articular swelling and erythema present, localized or diffuse)
         (sign
            (liver-gross contour abnormal ((liver contour description: distorted-or-
            asymmetrical))))
         (lab1 (antimitochondrial-antibody-titer increased))
         (lab4 (fibrosis without loss of hepatic lobular architecture present
            ((degree or amount slight) (pattern of hepatic fibrosis periportal)))
            (piecemeal necrosis of liver present))))
   (Characteristic findings ((lab2 (antigen-HBsAg positive))))))

Discussion

One of the reasons CPCS was developed was to provide a potential teaching tool for physicians in training, but at present CPCS has not yet been formally evaluated as a teaching tool. Nonetheless, CPCS did generate clinically consistent patient simulations, given the limited domain from which diseases were chosen.

Some expert systems have been developed that allow users to ask the expert system why a given conclusion was made, or why a given question was being asked.[8] This querying capability seems to be an essential part of assessing the functioning of a given expert system. However, some expert systems do not currently have that capability, yet they function at an appropriate level of expertness. For example, the QMR system allows users to explore its knowledge base and lets the user discover (by "critiquing a disease") why given questions are asked. The INTERNIST-1 system does not have such a capability. With its extensive knowledge of causal information, the CPCS system, if queried appropriately, is able to provide reasons (at a "deeper level" than QMR) why each item was chosen as being present in the simulated patient. The ability of CPCS to explain its choices was not implemented though. It is the author's opinion that if the knowledge base can be used to generate consistent patient cases that are indistinguishable from real patient information, which is converted to the vocabulary of the knowledge base by a human, that alone is a sufficient criterion for demonstrating that the knowledge base is of sufficient depth, causally speaking, to represent clinical reality.

Our results suggest a new method for evaluating expert systems. The ability to use the knowledge base of a given expert system to generate simulations of situations that are in the expert system's domain is another way in which a knowledge base can be used and explored. This exploration could discover gaps in the knowledge base domain that would be undiscovered in more straightforward use of the system. For example, the CPCS knowledge base was not conceived in its present form; this form grew out of an exploration of earlier versions (the INTERNIST-1/QMR format) that were inadequate in their ability to simulate patient cases. As inadequacies were discovered, the knowledge base was engineered to as accurately as possible contain information that resolved these inadequacies. The end result was a knowledge base with a sufficient level of information that resulted in adequate simulation of patient cases.

Another of the insights gained by the workers on this project was that representing knowledge to a causally sufficient level of detail requires a tremendous effort. From the effort involved in converting the existing INTERNIST-1/QMR liver diseases to the CPCS format, it is estimated that it would take approximately 250 person-years to convert all of the knowledge base to the CPCS structure. An area currently being investigated is a determination of which parts of the CPCS format for knowledge representation are crucial to achieve a sufficient degree of causal modeling. If this determination can be made, there is hope that by using those crucial areas of knowledge representation a method can be developed for capturing knowledge that does not require such a massive effort. However, because the final format of CPCS knowledge representation evolved as inadequacies were discovered, we may find that a less complex form does not exist that still maintains a sufficient level of causal information.

Developers of expert systems and their knowledge bases should make assessments of the following: the type of information needed for the knowledge base (by querying or simulation), the depth of representation necessary to achieve the desired performance, and the technologic and logistic limits of achieving that representation. The real question, then, is not whether causal reasoning can be done in expert systems or how causality in expert systems can be represented, but how we might represent causality to sufficient depth to provide functional improvement in the behavior of an expert system at a cost affordable in time and money.

Acknowledgments. Original development of CPCS was funded by National Library of Medicine New Investigator Award R23 LM 03589. The development of INTERNIST-1 was funded by the Division of Research Resources (R24 RR 01101) and the National Library of Medicine (R01 LM 03710). The development of QMR is funded by the CAMDAT Foundation of Farmington, Connecticut, the Department of Medicine of the University of Pittsburgh, and the National Library of Medicine (Research Career Development Award LM K04-00084).

References

1. Miller RA, Pople HE Jr, Myers JD: INTERNIST-1: an experimental computer-based diagnostic consultant for general internal medicine. N Engl J Med 307:468, 1982.
2. Patil RS, Szolovits P, Schwartz WB: Modeling knowledge of the patient in acid-base and electrolyte disorders. p. 191. In Szolovits P (ed): Artificial Intelligence in Medicine. AAAS Symposium Series. Boulder, CO: Westview Press, 1982.
3. Blois MS: Information and Medicine—The Nature of Medical Descriptions. Berkeley: University of California Press, 1984.
4. Pople HE, Myers JD, Miller RA: DIALOG: a model of diagnostic logic for internal medicine. p. 848. In: Proceedings of the Fourth International Joint Conference on Artificial Intelligence. Cambridge, MA: MIT Artificial Intelligence Laboratory Publications, 1975.
5. Miller RA, Masarie FE, Myers JD: Quick Medical Reference (QMR) for diagnostic assistance. MD Comput 3:34, 1986.
6. Miller RA, McNeil MA, Challinor SM, Masarie FE, Myers JD: The INTERNIST-1/QUICK MEDICAL REFERENCE project—status report. West J Med 145:816, 1986 (Medical Informatics: Special Issue).

7. Masarie FE, Miller RA, Myers JD: INTERNIST-1 properties: representing common sense and good medical practice in a computerized medical knowledge base. Comput Biomed Res 18:458, 1985.
8. Shortliffe EH: Computer-Based Medical Consultations: MYCIN. Artificial Intelligence Series. New York: Elsevier Computer Science Library, 1976.

9
Modeling and Encoding Clinical Causal Relations in a Medical Knowledge Base

Robert L. Blum

As research in artificial intelligence in medicine (AIM) has progressed, it has become increasingly apparent that in order to create computers that emulate the best human diagnosticians and clinicians, it is necessary to endow those computers with much if not all the knowledge that expert clinicians use. One category of knowledge that is critical to clinical reasoning is that of causal relations (CRs). Some examples of medical CRs follow. (1) Anxiety may cause insomnia. (2) The contracting left ventricle gives rise to flow of blood. (3) Penicillin may kill some strains of *Escherichia coli* in the urine. CRs may interrelate a diversity of objects at many levels of detail: clinical, systemic, cellular, and biochemical levels.

Before CRs can be encoded into a computer's knowledge base, it is necessary to have an adequate means of representing or modeling the various aspects of a CR in the computer. AIM researchers,[1] following the general methods of AI, have largely employed a modeling method called predicate calculus in their attempts to incorporate knowledge of CRs into machines for medical diagnosis.

In contrast to this AI work, another method for modeling CRs has been under development by biostatisticians, psychologists, and econometricians.[2] It is the method of path analysis and multivariate linear models.

In the course of our research we have developed a form for the representation of CRs that combines aspects of both these intellectual schools. The primary purpose of this report is to introduce some important features of this representation and to show some of the tasks it performs in the RX Project, described below.

RX Project: Automated Study and Incorporation of Causal Relations

Before presenting our method for representing CRs, it is helpful to know the research context in which it was elaborated. Our research project, called the RX Project, was begun in 1978 and is a multidisciplinary research effort whose purpose is to develop techniques for deriving various types of medical knowledge from clinical data bases. To date, we have been concerned exclusively with the detection and study of CRs in our data bases and with their subsequent incorporation and use by the program.

Specifically, the objectives of the project are to (1) increase the validity of CRs derivable from large time-oriented clinical data bases, (2) develop methods for providing intelligent assistance with the task of testing hypothesized CRs against a data base, and (3) study methods for automating the process of discovering CRs. The RX Project was definitively described by Blum[3] and was later summarized by Blum.[4]

The RX methodology for deriving possible causal relations from a clinical data base employs the following components: a knowledge base, a discovery module, a study module, a statistical package, and a clinical data base. In brief, the system works as follows. The discovery module examines relevant subsets of the data base to generate an ordered list of causal hypotheses. These hypotheses, of the form "A causes B," are sequentially examined by the study module. The study module uses the knowledge base to generate a comprehensive epidemiologic study design of the hypothesis. This study design is then tested on the statistical package using the entire data base. The results are passed back to the study module for interpretation. If the results are medically important as well as statistically significant, they are written as a new, machine-readable causal relation into the knowledge base. The process of automated study design (Fig. 9.1) makes use of previously "learned" causal relations.

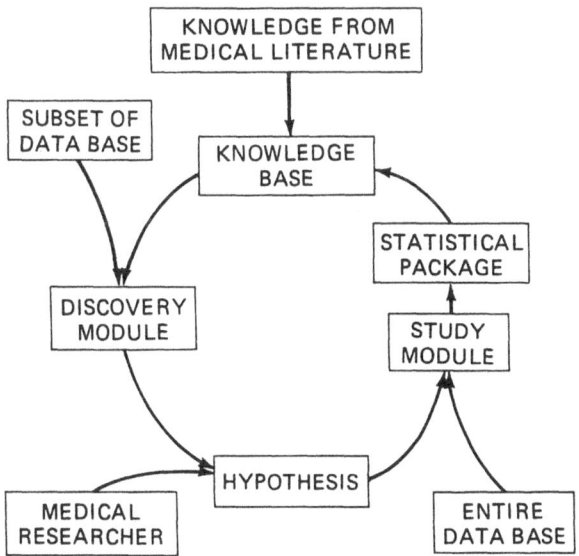

Figure 9.1. Discovery/confirmation/incorporation cycle of RX.

The clinical data base we use is a 1700-patient subset of the ARAMIS data base[5,6] occupying 15,000 pages. Medical CRs the program "discovered" using a small preliminary subset are described elsewhere.[4] (Most of the discovered CRs were previously described in the medical literature.)

Design Criteria for the Representation of Causal Relations for RX

The form in which we have chosen to represent CRs in RX has been strongly influenced by the necessity of capturing detailed information on them and of using that information for the subsequent study and confirmation of other CRs.

The principal objective of the RX Project is to derive and incorporate detailed knowledge of causal relations from large time-oriented data bases. This knowledge is stored interchangeably with knowledge entered into the medical knowledge base from the medical literature. It is necessary that the representation of CRs be sufficiently rich to enable capturing information on magnitude, frequency, and variability of effect, distribution in a patient population, mathematic form, clinical setting, validity or reliability, and evidential basis.

Although the representation we have designed enables most of these aspects to be encoded in machine-readable form, the most important motivating factor when designing an adequate representation is the tasks for which the encoded information will be used. The only task we describe here is the study module's use of CRs for creating a study design for a causal hypothesis. This task requires information on the intensity of causal links, their mathematic form, their distribution across patients, and their clinical setting.

A critical step in the design of a study by the RX study module involves selection of the set of known clinical events that may confound or bias the results of a study. This set of events is known as the set of confounding variables. The control of confounding variables is an essential step in the design of studies using routine health care data. A confounding variable is one that may affect both the causal variable and the effect variable of interest. The objective of control is to attempt to isolate the relation from spurious causal influence. For example, if A is a drug and B is a side effect of interest, we want to control for diseases that affect both A and B.

The task of demonstrating that a causal relation is nonspurious is by far the most difficult task in deriving CRs from large clinical data bases. Unfortunately, the confounding variables may exert their influence indirectly, as shown in Figure 9.2. Here there are four confounding variables: F, G, H, and D. If we were to examine only the list of variables that directly affect B, however, we would find only F and E. The node E is not a confounding variable, as it is known not to affect A.

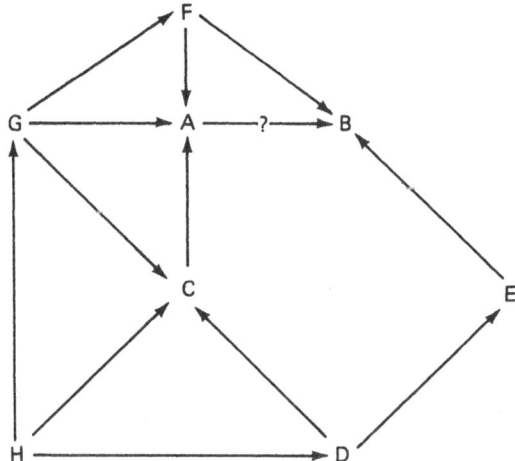

Figure 9.2. Confounding variables.

To determine the set of confounding variables for the hypothesis "A causes B," the study module uses a function called confounding-variables to traverse a directed graph whose arcs are CRs. The function determines the set of all nodes that may have medically significant effects (greater than some magnitude) on both A and B for a given clinical setting.

The study module controls for only a subset of the confounding variables called the causal dominators. This subset is defined as the smallest subset through which all known causal influence on both A and B must flow. In Figure 9.2 this set = {F D}.

Representation of Causal Relations in the RX Knowledge Base

In brief, CRs are represented as labeled arcs in a directed graph in which the nodes are frames. For the sake of this discussion we assume that X is a causal node and Y is an effect node. They are connected by a CR whose components are described in detail. We specify both the X and Y objects as having real-valued intensities. In other words, in this discussion we model them as real-valued variables. We assume the following relation between their intensities:

$$Y(t + \text{tau}) = bf[X(t)] = e$$

That is, Y's value at time t + tau is linearly related to some function of Xs value at time t (+ an error term e). We further assume that the relation is causal. That is, a change in X of one unit induces a change in Y of $bf[1]$ after tau time units. X is assumed to cause Y in the probabilistic sense that it accounts for some of its variance. In the usual path analysis or regression model, we could estimate the parameters of the model by using a data base of pairs of measurements of X and Y. The estimate of greatest importance is the unstandardized regression coefficient b. If b is significantly different from zero, we then posit that X causes Y.

The basic information conveyed by the model is that an increase in X by one unit causes a change in Y by b units, where b is the unstandardized coefficient of Y on X. Labeled with just these regression coefficients, a simple directed graph can be set up to represent chains of causality as below.

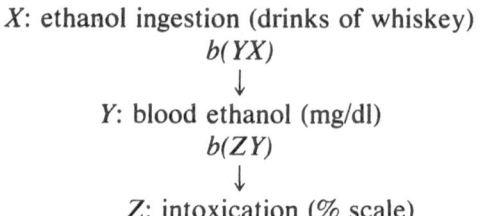

Although this representation captures some information about the intensity of the relations, it neglects several other key aspects.

A causal link in the RX knowledge base is composed of seven components: intensity, distribution, direction, functional-form, setting, validity, and evidence.

In what follows we have assumed that both the causal variable and the effect variable connected by this causal relation are real-valued. In our future work we intend to generalize this formalism so that binary and rank-valued variables may also be arbitrarily connected. The meaning of each of these seven components is summarized below:

Intensity: the expected change in the effect given in the cause, expressed as an unstandardized regression coefficient.

Distribution: the distribution of the intensity of the effect across patients.

Direction: increases or decreases.

Setting: the circumstances under which the causal relation was derived, encoded as a Boolean expression with time-dependent predicates.

Functional form: the complete mathematic model relating Y to X, encoded in an algebraic language.

Validity: the state of proof of the causal relation on a 1 to 10 scale: 1 means highly tentative, 10 means beyond reasonable doubt.

Evidence: a summary of the evidence on which the relation is based: either literature citations or a summary of the study performed by the study module.

In the RX study module the intensity and the direction components are derived from the fitted regression model that is stored in machine-readable form as the functional-form component.

The distribution component records the density function of the estimated regression coefficients across patients. In other words, this component enables us to record the varying intensities with which a population of patients exhibits the effect of interest. This capability for encoding unexplained variation in an effect is an important aspect of our representation scheme. This density function is encoded by storing the mass under ten contiguous regions of the curve. The choice of the nine cut points is based on prior medical knowledge of the effect variable.

The setting component allows the explicit inclusion of the setting in which the causal relation is believed to be true. For relations that have been empirically derived by the study module, the setting component encodes the inclusion and exclusion criteria that were used to select time intervals from patient records for study. In English a typical setting might read "between 2 months and 6 months after myocardial infarction but not during an episode of congestive heart failure." This statement is stored as a logical expression with time-dependent functions, e.g., (concurrent (after myocardial infarction 2 months 6 months) (not (during congestive heart failure))).

The validity of a causal relation is represented simply as an integer from 1 to 10, from lowest reliability to highest. The scale is, of course, arbitrary but captures an important dimension of causal knowledge. In the current study module the validity is derived from a set of tables where the rows and columns of the tables are "statistical significance" (p value) and "medical significance." Medical significance is simply based on the relative magnitude of the size of the effect. In other words, it asks, "Is the size of the effect sufficient to merit inclusion in the knowledge base?" (Large studies can yield effects that are statistically but not medically significant.) The choice among the tables depends on the study design used for deriving the effect. Longitudinal study designs merit tables with higher validities than do cross-sectional designs.

Linear Models Versus Predicate Calculus

The representation for CRs presented here was strongly influenced by the methods of linear models, multivariate analysis, and path analysis. This body of theory has largely been developed and applied by psychologists, economists, and biologists. Excellent reviews are available.[2,7] In contrast, workers in the field of artificial intelligence have largely used representations based on predicate calculus and other systems of logic. Many[8–10] have largely been applied to the simulation and understanding of mechanical and electrical devices.

Why have multivariate linear models been used for certain applications and predicate calculus models for others? The answer is profound and important: Linear models capture crucial features of natural systems; predicate calculus captures crucial features of artifacts.

Natural systems are inherently probabilistic. Medical phenomena, at least at the clinical level, are typically indeterminate. This probabilistic character arises from at least four sources: (1) the inherently probabilistic nature of the component phenomena (at all levels of detail) that comprise the working human body; (2) our inability as observers to accurately measure these phenomena in a given patient; (3) the variability of effects across patients; and (4) the inadequacy of current biologic theory as a basis for explanation. The role of probability in models of causality was lucidly discussed by Suppes.[11]

Capturing this variability of clinical phenomena in a sufficiently detailed manner to allow its subsequent scientific analysis dictates that detailed quantitative information on the intensities of effects and their variation be captured in the representation. It is largely what has motivated adoption of multivariate linear models and extensions to them. In RX we start with detailed quantitative data in the data base. We have tried to preserve as much of that detail as possible in the statistical summaries that comprise the data in the CRs.

Although the preoccupation of most AI researchers with predicate calculus may be justified by its adequacy for modeling mechanical devices, it may be found lacking when used in programs that perform medical diagnosis, e.g., INTERNIST or PIP.[1] For example, if two diseases can coexist and both can raise the serum sodium level, INTERNIST can attribute hypernatremia only to either disease, not both, and PIP assumes that both diseases may have caused it but cannot make use of the actual sodium value to decide if the two diseases might have co-occurred. Only by incorporation of detailed numerically based models is there any hope of correctly quantitating concurrent causal influences in programs that purport to do expert medical reasoning.

Conclusion

A simple representation for CRs appropriate for modeling some aspects of clinical medicine has been shown. The model distinguishes two general categories of attributes of CRs: (1) those describing the particular causal phenomenon per se, and (2) those pertaining to the extent of belief in the existence of the phenomenon. The phenomenon itself is described by attributes encoding its intensity, distribution in a population of patients, its functional form (or "dose–response" curve), and its clinical setting. Belief concerning the phenomenon's existence is encoded by a validity attribute (simple 1 to 10 scale) and an evidence attribute (summarizing the supporting evidence). The representation was most strongly influenced by the methods of multivariate linear models and path analysis.

The usefulness of linear models in representations of clinical CRs was seen to arise from several key features that distinguish natural systems from manmade systems. Knowledge of natural systems is fundamentally probabilistic because of (1) irreducible indeterminism in the component processes, (2) difficulty of accurately measuring all relevant variables, (3) variation among individuals in a population, and (4) inadequate scientific theory.

Given that detailed quantitative information is occasionally needed in medical AI programs, how does the user or the program avoid being bogged down in needless complexity? The solution is to maintain detailed information in the knowledge base and to translate it, as needed, to appropriately simplified levels. Linear models, in particular, may be automatically simplified into predicate calculus forms (but not vice versa).

In the future we want to extend the representational method presented here by including the following: (1) variables at all measurement levels (binary, categorical, rank, real); (2) diverse nonlinear forms; (3) interactions of variables; (4) different link types (causal versus associational versus definitional). In addition, we want to investigate formal methods for combining evidence from multiple sources.

Acknowledgments. Funding for this research was provided by the National Center for Health Services Research (grant HS-04389) and by the National Library of Medicine (grant LM-03370). Computation facilities were provided by SUMEX-AIM through NIH grant RR-00785 from the Biotechnology Resources Program. Clinical data were obtained from the American Rheumatism Association Medical Information System (ARAMIS), which is sponsored by NIH grants AM-21393 and HS-03802.

References

1. Szolovits P (ed): Artificial Intelligence in Medicine. Boulder, CO: Westview Press, 1982.
2. Bentler PM: Multivariate analysis with latent variables: causal modeling. Annu Rev Psychol 31:419, 1980.
3. Blum RL: Discovery and Representation of Causal Relationships from a Large Time-Oriented Database: The RX Project (Vol. 19 in the Medical Informatics Series, edited by D. Lindberg and P. Reichertz). New York: Springer Verlag, 1982.
4. Blum RL: Discovery, confirmation, and incorporation of causal relationships from a large time-oriented database: the RX project. Comput Biomed Res 15:164, 1982.
5. Fries JF, McShane DJ: ARAMIS: a national chronic disease data bank system. p. 798. In: Proceedings of the Third Annual Symposium on Computer Applications in Medical Care. Washington DC: IEEE, 1979.
6. McShane D, Harlow A, Kraines R, Fries J: TOD: a software system for the ARAMIS data bank. Computer 12:34, 1979.
7. Heise D: Path Analysis. New York: Wiley, 1979.
8. De Kleer J, Brown JS: Mental models of physical mechanisms and their acquisition. In Anderson J (ed): Cognitive Skills and Their Acquisition. Hillsdale, NJ: Erlbaum, 1981.

9. Rieger C, Grinberg M: The declarative representation and procedural simulation of causality in physical mechanisms. p. 250. In: Proceedings of the 5th International Joint Conference on Artificial Intelligence. Boston, MA: IJCAI, 1977.
10. Rieger C, Grinberg M: A system of cause-effect representation and simulation for computer-aided design. p. 299. In Latombe JC (ed): Artificial Intelligence and Pattern Recognition in Computer-Aided Design. Amsterdam: North Holland, 1978.
11. Suppes P: A Probabilistic Theory of Causality. Amsterdam: North Holland, 1970.

10
Computational Model of Reasoning from the Clinical Literature

Glenn D. Rennels, Edward H. Shortliffe,
Frank E. Stockdale, and Perry L. Miller

Artificial intelligence research has increasingly emphasized the advantages of representing more fundamental knowledge about the problem domain than, for instance, a set of weighted links between observable findings and diagnostic hypotheses. Much of this work seeks to flesh out the causal models underlying diagnostic reasoning and to represent those models ("deep models") in an expert system to help drive its reasoning process. For example, an electronic circuit or a functioning human body is modeled, and computer programs are designed to search for causal explanations of malfunction.[1-3] Planning medical management has not been as fully investigated, but several projects are currently exploring the notion that causal models of human pathophysiology can drive the analysis of medical management, for instance by simulating the effects of perturbing homeostasis in various ways.[4]

When these models mirror a manufactured device (e.g., an electronic circuit), causal models may indeed provide a sound basis for advice systems. In empiric sciences such as biomedicine, however, these models are secondary constructions, derived from experimental evidence. A medical example is breast cancer. Biologic models of breast cancer are an unreliable basis for therapy planning, and the physician's reasoning must be directly grounded in the primary sources of experimental evidence (clinical trial publications).

Clinicians are well aware that good medical practice depends on keeping up to date with the clinical literature. To use this literature most effectively, a physician must critically assess these studies in the context of a particular patient and decide in what ways the experimental trial is relevant to the case at hand. Indeed, this skill of recalling the key studies and evaluating how well those results apply to the patient is a process learned and practiced every day by teams of residents on "rounds." A computer system that fails to use this fundamental knowledge may therefore not fully capture the decision-making process of many medical domains. Nevertheless, there

© 1986 by the Institute of Electrical and Electronics Engineers, Inc. Reprinted with permission from the *Proceedings of the 10th Annual Symposium on Computer Applications in Medical Care*, Washington, D.C., Oct 25–26, pp. 373–380.

has been little or no research on the design of computer systems that reason explicitly from clinical studies to provide decision support for physicians.

This chapter describes a computer program in development, named Roundsman, that draws on structured representations of the clinical literature to critique plans for medical management. The goal of the Roundsman project is to model the process of reasoning from the clinical literature. There are many medical domains in which such reasoning dominates. It is therefore important to explore how a machine might assist a clinician in this literature-based reasoning process.

The Roundsman project differs substantially from causal modeling in that there is no desire to model a "device" and its function but, rather, to model the structure of experimental evidence and its interpretation for decision-making. In medical terms, it is not pathophysiologic knowledge that is represented, but knowledge about experimental trials and their relevance to a particular patient.

Nature of the Problem

How does a physician reason from the clinical literature? To gain insight into this question, the Roundsman project began with a period of informal protocol analysis. Previous work in medical protocol analysis has investigated diagnostic reasoning[5,6] and has been particularly oriented toward causal models.[7] A senior oncologist at Stanford University Medical Center was asked to "think aloud" as he formulated management plans for primary breast cancer. These sessions were tape-recorded and later analyzed. By varying the clinical studies the oncologist could draw on, it was possible to examine how a particular study contributed to the reasoning process, and how a study's role changed as additional studies were added to the "library." We were particularly interested in how the oncologist's clinical judgment affected the interpretation of statistical results and of the study as a whole.

Analysis of these transcripts suggested several organizational views. Here we discuss one of these views (a *publication-centered view*) and its corresponding system design issues.

With the publication-centered view, critical readers embed the results of a clinical study in a matrix of contextual details "attached" to a particular clinical study. These contextual details help interpret the meaning of the study's statistical results. Such details include: (1) What type of patients seek care at the hospital where the research was done? To use the study as a basis for treatment, a physician must assess the differences between the study population and the patient in question and decide whether those differences are likely to influence outcome. (2) What is the track record of the author? Have the previously published results been reproducible by other teams? (3) How qualified are the allied specialties that are involved in patient care but that are not the subject of investigation, e.g., postoperative nursing care? (4) What are the exact technical details for the treatments being compared (e.g., two studies may compare the same drugs, but the dose and dosing schedules might differ)? Before the study can be used as a basis for therapy planning, a physician must consider if the technical approach used in the study differed significantly from the approach now planned. (5) How sophisticated is the biostatistical analysis?

An awareness of these contextual details allows physicians to decide how relevant the study is to their particular patient and treatment plan. The importance of this issue is seen in the examples provided below and in the design of a *distance metric*, as discussed later in the chapter and described more fully elsewhere.[8]

These contextual details overlay the study's experimental design and results. The design and results may have significant complexity themselves and frequently require analysis when assessing the study's relevance. For example, longitudinal, prospective comparisons of deliberate intervention[9] compare one therapy group to another, control group; optimally, these groups are studied in parallel. Nevertheless, one of the most important sources of medical information has been the "case series" study, in which controls are external to the study (and therefore not formally matched at all).

Another dimension of design complexity concerns stratification. Patients are often sorted into strata according to variables thought to influence significantly their response to therapy. Results are then presented by stratum. Physicians can weed out many irrelevant tables and charts from the report if they can determine which stratum applies best to their patient. Even here, however, the critical reader exercises clinical judgment. For example, if the strata were constructed after treatment ("poststratification"), one must assess the investigator's intent: Was the stratification motivated by genuine clinical concerns, or was it the product of a "fishing expedition" for a stratum that was statistically significant?

This publication-centered model, in which knowledge is structured around studies as distinct entities, also allows the natural representation of inter-study knowledge. For example, study A might have had an irregularity in the experimental design that left some doubt as to the generalizability of the main conclusions. Study B, published some time later, might demonstrate that the irregularity makes no difference, thus strengthening the principal conclusions of study A, even though it might have investigated a different question.

There are other ways one might structure this knowledge. The remainder of this section, however, focuses on four design goals of Roundsman's publication-centered implementation:

1. The computer system's data structures must reflect the publication-centered view. In particular, the system's critique of a treatment pro-

posal for a particular patient must spring from declarative representations of one or more study's experimental design and observed
outcomes.
2. There must be convenient ways to represent knowledge about the contextual details mentioned earlier, many of which are the subjective
clinical judgments of the domain expert.
3. These contextual details must influence system performance in a sub-
stantive way. Ideally, the system discusses the basic statistical results
with the same priority and in the same manner as the domain expert.
4. The system must address clinical concerns in a realistic way and communicate in English well enough that clinical practitioners and biostatisticians can evaluate the potential of this approach to decision
support.

Roundsman System: Examples

The Roundsman program contains a library of clinical studies, each of
which is represented as a separate data structure. They are not full-text
copies of articles but, instead, are high-level representations of the study's
features. Examples of Roundsman using these studies to critique a physician's plan are given below. Each example includes a verbatim transcript
of Roundsman's current output.

To use Roundsman, the physician first describes the patient (e.g., age
45, stage II breast cancer, premenopausal) and proposes a therapy choice
(e.g., surgical wide excision followed by adjuvant radiotherapy). Roundsman produces a prose critique of the plan in light of the study. This critique
is assembled dynamically, tailored to the particular patient, treatment decision, and clinical study(ies). The prose is generated by Roundsman's
TEXTNET facility, an adaptation of Miller's PROSENET,[10] based on the
augmented transition net formalism.

In each example Roundsman is critiquing a proposal for the surgical
management of a particular patient's breast cancer. Because the critiques
are rich in clinical detail, it must be reemphasized that Roundsman is
currently a research project. These critiques are an important first step
toward providing a new type of computer-based decision support, but
they *cannot* be used as advice for clinical decisions at this time. Indeed,
the trained clinician may notice comments that are clinically controversial
or possibly incorrect. Further research and development are needed, as
well as more intensive collaboration with the medical experts in the domain.

Each example consists in: (1) a statement of the clinical context (a
description of the patient and the physician's treatment proposal); (2) a
verbatim transcript of Roundsman's critique of one particular study in
light of that clinical context; and (3) a discussion of certain aspects of the

example critique. For each clinical context, Roundsman usually selected three to five studies for discussion. Ultimately, Roundsman will consider the overall impact of a group of studies; at present, however, Roundsman critiques each relevant study serially. The output in these examples is typical of Roundsman's performance; and the only "selection" involved was making sure that the examples included biomedical reports with different experimental designs, from more than one time period, and that the examples show how a study's critique changes for different clinical contexts.

Example 1

Clinical Context.

1. A 45-year-old premenopausal woman with tumor size T1a, axillary lymph nodes N1a, unknown axillary node histology (which cannot be known until after surgery), and no metastases
2. Treatment proposal: surgical wide excision (and axillary dissection) plus adjuvant radiotherapy plus adjuvant chemotherapy if axillary node histology is subsequently positive

Roundsman's Critique. The following verbatim transcript shows Roundsman discussing the relevance of a publication by Fisher et al.[11]

Fisher85a was a randomized, controlled trial conducted at multiple NSABP centers. Subjects were assigned to verified wide excision with axillary dissection and adjuvant radiotherapy (N = 373) or the alternative therapy of verified wide excision with axillary dissection (N = 358). For patients who underwent the first protocol the proportion free of ipsilateral breast recurrence at five years was equal to 0.9, overall survival at five years turned out to be 0.91 and recurrence-free survival at five years was 0.81. Under the second protocol the proportion free of ipsilateral breast recurrence at five years turned out to be 0.77, overall survival at five years was 0.9 and recurrence-free survival at five years was equal to 0.68.

Are these results relevant to your patient? It is encouraging that, first, the adjuvant modality you propose was specified for this study as well (chemotherapy given if axillary nodes are path. positive). Second, this study population is quite similar to your patient (the women in this group had T sizes ranging up to T2a but excision margins were verified free of tumor). We suspect it makes little difference that the intervention was somewhat nonstandard (they did not radiate supraclavicular nodes). More troublesome is that the study population was probably in a better prognostic stratum than your patient (this study stratum was defined by negative axillary node histology; about 40% of clinical stage I patients like yours will have positive histology).

What is the validity of the data? It helps that first, the investigator is reliable (the NSABP trials are first-rate, e.g., participating physicians must be certified by Fisher). Second, controls were randomly assigned. The results are weakened because one of their outcomes was a bit nonstandard (recurrence in the ipsilateral breast was NOT counted as a local recurrence).

More than one outcome type is reported, but strictly on the basis of five-year results in recurrence-free survival, your suggested therapy seems best (although not all results agree). The close fit of your patient, considered together with the excellent methodology, probably would not alter that statistical conclusion. The first protocol mentioned (which is close to your proposed plan) appears to be the better one.

Example 1 illustrates several reasons why the clinical literature is an interesting problem area for employing computer-based decision support.

Complexity of experimental design: This trial (NSABP protocol 6) compares three interventions in parallel: (1) total mastectomy; (2) excision ("lumpectomy"); and (3) excision plus radiation. In certain subsets of each group, chemotherapy was used. Several endpoints were reported: overall survival, recurrence-free survival, and ipsilateral breast recurrence. For the physician requesting this consultation, Roundsman has decided to highlight a comparison of intervention arms 2 and 3. Proper analysis of the results is complicated by the fact that the patients used to compute the results of intervention 2 are not the same when interventions 1 and 2 are compared as when interventions 3 and 2 are compared (as is discussed more fully in example 2). This design complexity has a domain-specific motivation that is of more interest to oncologists than computer scientists. The important point is that even in just presenting the first paragraph Roundsman has already done a significant amount of work for the physician by sifting through the numerous interventions, subsets of patients, and endpoints in order to present selective portions of a complex body of experimental evidence. Next comes Roundsman's principal focus: the further subjective assessment of the relevance of those selective portions to the physician's clinical case.

Clinical details of the study: Although certain clinical details are crucial to intelligent assessment of the study for clinical purposes, it is practically impossible for a physician to recall these details months or years after reading the article. The cost of refreshing these details is a line-by-line reading of a lengthy technical article. For example, certain clinical conditions had to exist before chemotherapy was given (paragraph 2), several tumor (T) sizes were allowed in this group of women studied, but excision margins were verified free of tumor (paragraph 2), supraclavicular nodes (i.e., lymph nodes located above the collarbone) were not exposed to radiation (paragraph 2), and the definition of "local recurrence" excluded recurrences in the breast that had the original tumor (paragraph 3). Thus Roundsman brings to light certain clinical details that may help the physician use this experimental evidence for his purposes.

Relevance of clinical detail to the physician making a particular management decision: The second and third paragraphs not only offer subjective judgments about which clinical details of the study should be explicitly juxtaposed against the physician's patient and treatment decision, but in addition offer subjective judgments about the *importance* of any mismatch when using the study to discuss the management problem under consideration. For example, the fact that the physician also plans to use chemotherapy if the axillary node histology turns out to be positive (paragraph 2) makes it easier to say that the report can provide some support for this management decision. Irradiation of supraclavicular nodes is judged to be a minor detail whatever the physician chooses to do.

Example 2

Example 2 shows how Roundsman's critique of Fisher85a (the study discussed in example 1) changes when the physician's patient is different.

Clinical Context.

1. A 45-year-old premenopausal woman with tumor size T1a, axillary lymph node status N1b, unknown axillary node histology, and no metastases
2. Treatment proposal: surgical wide excision (and axillary dissection) plus adjuvant radiotherapy plus adjuvant chemotherapy if axillary node histology is subsequently positive

Roundsman's Critique.

Fisher85a was a randomized, controlled trial performed by investigators at multiple NSABP centers. Patients were randomized to wide excision (& axillary dissection) and adjuvant radiotherapy and adjuvant chemotherapy (N = 229) or another protocol which was total mastectomy (& axillary dissection) and adjuvant chemotherapy (N = 224). For patients who underwent the first protocol the overall survival at five years turned out to be 0.75 and recurrence-free survival at five years was equal to 0.58. Under the second protocol the overall survival at five years was 0.66 and recurrence-free survival at five years was equal to 0.58.

How do these data apply to your patient? We are not particularly concerned that the intervention was somewhat nonstandard (they did not radiate supraclavicular nodes). More troublesome is that first, there were modifications to one intervention (in the excision arm, women with positive margins received total mastectomy, but remained in the "excision" group). Second, the study population was in a worse prognostic stratum compared to your patient (this study stratum was defined by positive axillary node histology; about 40% of clinical stage II patients like yours will have negative histology).

How much confidence can we have in the experimental results? It's good to see that, first, the investigator is reliable (the NSABP trials are first-rate, e.g., participating physicians must be certified by Fisher). Second, controls were randomly assigned. The results are weakened because one of their outcomes was a bit nonstandard (recurrence in the ipsilateral breast was NOT counted as a local recurrence).

Looking selectively at five-year results in recurrence-free survival, those two interventions look equivalent (the other results generally agree). The "relevance" problems detailed above, considered together with the excellent methodology probably would not alter that statistical conclusion. Consequently, a choice between these two approaches might be made on the basis of morbidity (cosmesis, etc.) rather than cure.

In example 2, Roundsman's critique has changed in several ways from that shown in example 1.

Dealing with the complexity of the experimental design: The patient in example 2 has worse disease than the woman considered in example 1. This patient has stage II breast cancer, and it is more controversial if excision is a safer surgical approach for her disease than for the woman in example 1. Consequently, in example 2 Roundsman chooses to focus its discussion on a comparison of a different surgical approach, rather than a comparison of the omission or addition of irradiation (as in example 1). As mentioned earlier, Fisher85a studied three interventions in parallel, so for this example Roundsman has presented evidence concerning total mastectomy versus wide excision.

Relevance of clinical detail to the physician making a particular management decision: As mentioned in the discussion of example 1, the patients used to determine the results of intervention 2 are not the same when interventions 1 and 2 are compared as when interventions 3 and 2 are compared. Understanding this point requires attention to clinical detail: The Fisher85a protocol specified that women entered into the excision arm *must* have the margins of their excision verified free of tumor. If margins are *not* free, the woman went on to have a total mastectomy. For the analysis of the excision group versus the total mastectomy group, women who failed to have clear margins (and thus underwent total mastectomies) *were counted as members of the excision group.* Why? To exclude them would have biased the results: The total mastectomy group did not check excision margins; excluding unclear margins from the excision group would exclude women with bigger tumors, making the results look better than they should. This clinical detail is brought to the attention of the physician in sentence 3 of paragraph 2 in the critique just above.

One might then ask why this clinical detail was not mentioned in the critique in example 1? It was not done because when comparing "excision" versus "excision plus radiotherapy" (discussed in example 1), women who fail to have clean margins and therefore undergo total mastectomy are excluded from the count. The critique in example 1 need not concern the physician with clinical detail(s) of the study that do not have an impact on the clinical context currently being considered.

Example 3

Example 3 shows what a consultation with Roundsman would look like if the date were 1967. In order to do it, Roundsman is restricted to publications that appeared prior to 1968. Also, the date of the consultation (a system variable) is set to "1967." In 1967 total mastectomy was being advocated by some physicians, but it was a controversial management decision: The consensus was that doing less than a radical mastectomy endangered the life of a woman with breast cancer.

In examples 1 and 2 Roundsman discussed a randomized, controlled study. Example 3 shows Roundsman critiquing a clinical study that used nonrandomized internal controls. The publication discussed in this example[12] appeared in the literature when radical mastectomy was the standard of care and surgical excision was used by only a small minority of surgeons.

Clinical Context (year 1967).

1. A 45-year-old premenopausal woman whose clinical examination reveals tumor size T1a, whose axillary nodes are thought to contain tumor (N1b), and who has no metastases
2. Treatment proposal: wide excision, axillary dissection, and adjuvant radiotherapy

Roundsman's Critique.

Peters employed non-randomized controls in a study conducted at Princess Margaret Hospital, Toronto. A set of patients who were treated by wedge resection and adjuvant radiotherapy (N = 94) is contrasted to a second therapy group: radical mastectomy and adjuvant radiotherapy (N = 247). In the group which received the first protocol the overall survival at five years was 0.76. For patients who underwent the second protocol the overall survival at five years turned out to be 0.72.

How well does the study generalize to your particular patient? We are not particularly concerned that one modality you propose may not be quite like what was done in the study ("wedge resection" here indicates excisional biopsy, quadrant resection, or any technique to excise the primary). More troublesome is that the study population was probably in a better prognostic stratum than your patient (the study used a pooled clinical stage I and II - so that's a slightly better prognostic group than your patient).

How much confidence can we have in the experimental results? The results are weakened because, first, choice of treatment was decided nonrandomly (nor were subjects and controls matched on prognostic parameters). Second, patients were accrued over a rather long period (this is a retrospective study of patients treated between 1935 and 1960). Third, this is a wide stratum (it would have been preferable to separate stages I and II).

Considering the reported observations and sample size (see introductory paragraph), those two interventions look equivalent. The small mismatch of your particular clinical situation, considered together with the large methodological weaknesses however, leads us to think that the results are indecisive for your purposes. Adhering to the standard of care (radical mastectomy) would probably be most appropriate.

In retrospect, the nearly equivalent proportions reported in paragraph 1 (above) have been borne out by later studies that compared mastectomy to excision (e.g., Fisher85a in examples 1 and 2). In this consultation, however, Roundsman is unable to confidently conclude that Peters67 provides enough support for the physician to deviate from more standard surgical approach (see last sentence of the concluding paragraph). The reasons for this lack of support are explained by Roundsman: the nonuniform nature of the intervention (paragraph 2), the broad stratum of patients lumped together for analysis (paragraph 2), the nonrandom experimental design (paragraph 3), and the long accrual period (paragraph 3).

System Design of Roundsman

This section provides an overview of the Roundsman system's flow of control and describes Roundsman's principal data structures.

Control

An outline of the steps taken by Roundsman when analyzing a case (Fig. 10.1) is provided below.

1. Establish the "decision context." The decision context includes information about the patient and the therapy the physician is proposing for that patient.
2. Focus on the class of questions most likely to interest the physician. It entails deciding what types of therapeutic intervention should be compared. For example, during one time period it might be more appropriate for the machine to first discuss the surgical procedure, whereas during another time period it would be more appropriate to first discuss the use (or omission) of adjuvant radiation with the proposed surgery. The need to establish an appropriate focus results because the clinical "consensus" changes over time.
3. Determine, for each study in the library, if it can provide experimental results concerning that class of questions. If so:
   a. Find the group (stratum) of patients within the study that most closely approximates the physician's patient.
   b. For that stratum, identify any experimental results following treatment with the interventions of interest (see step 2).

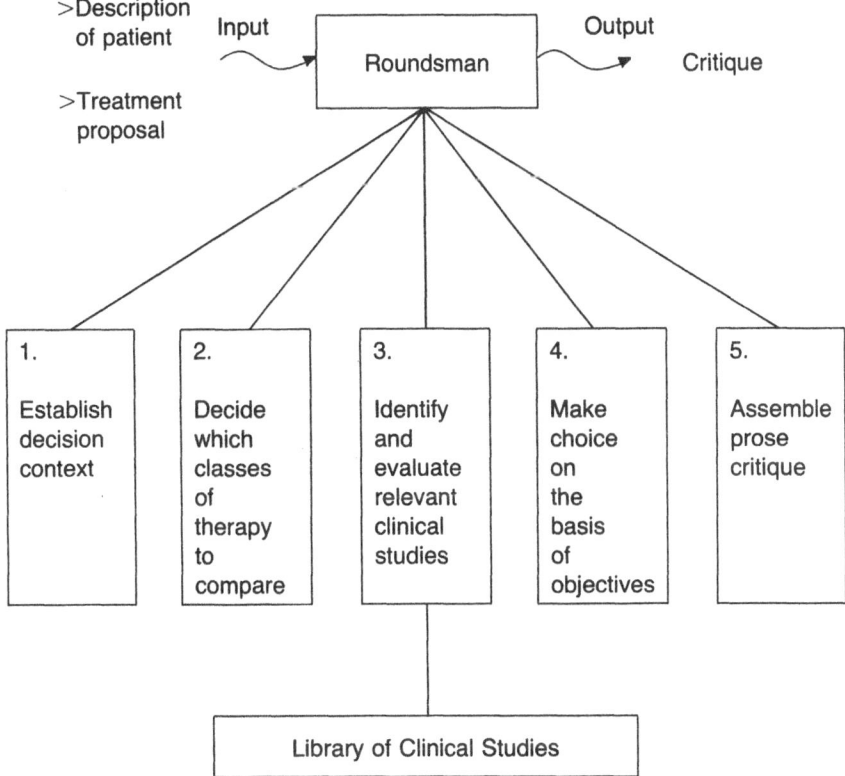

Figure 10.1. Flow of control in the Roundsman system.

    c. Assess the "distances" between the physician's decision context and the particulars of the clinical study. (This process is discussed more fully below when Roundsman's distance-metric and distance-estimator are described.)

    d. Return the study results as applied to the chosen stratum, together with the distance assessments, to higher level control functions in Roundsman. All this information is packaged in an object called a "datum-from-study."

4. Use the datum-from-study to compare alternative interventions on the basis of a model of choice and explanation.

5. Pass the conclusions of the system to a prose generation module that assembles a prose critique for the user.

Data Structures

The Roundsman system is organized around frame-based data structures. The most prominent of these data structures is the *study*. For example, the Peters77 study is one of 24 publications currently represented in Roundsman's "library." The heart of each study consists of strata (sets of the data structure *stratum*) and comparisons (sets of the data structure *comparison*), each of which is discussed below. In addition, each study contains certain descriptive information, e.g., the name of the institution where the research was carried out.

A stratum is a definition of the study population. Publications of clinical studies do not report data at the level of individual patients. Thus a stratum is not a collection of patients, as in a data base, but a summary description for a population. Consequently, the central component of each stratum is a population description, a data structure (not text strings) that can be interpreted by the machine. For example, one population description is shown:

POPULATION-DESCRIPTION with
    Clinical stage set = (I, II)
    T set   = (T0, T1a, T1b, T2a, T2b)
    N set   = (N0, N1a)
    Path N set = (unknown)
    M set   = (M0)
    Menopausal status set = (pre post)
    Age, lower-bound. = 20
    Age, upper-bound. = 80

This population description includes patients of varying tumor sizes (T0 through T2b), a narrow range of clinical node status (N0 and N1a), unknown axillary node pathology, no distant metastases (M0), and a wide age span.

In addition to strata, a key part of any study is the *comparison* object. Each comparison contains knowledge about an experiment comparing one therapeutic intervention against another. For example, one comparison from the Peters67 study is shown:

COMPARISON with
    Study ID   = Peters67
    Stratum ID   = 1
    Comparison ID = 1
    Intervention A = <pointer to an intervention>
    Intervention B = <pointer to an intervention>
    Sample size A = 203
    Sample size B = 609
    Outcome A   = <pointer to an outcome>
    Outcome B   = <pointer to an outcome>
    Standard error of difference = 0.056

This comparison encodes details about the *interventions* being compared, the stratum involved, and the *outcomes* that were measured. In addition, each comparison may identify the study it belongs to (with identifier "Peters67"). The comparison shown above (with integer identifier

1) might have outcomes pertaining to overall survival at 5 years, whereas comparison 2 might pertain to recurrence-free survival at 10 years. The motivation for placing this information into separate comparisons is not discussed here. Each of these components is, in turn, a data structure. For example, Roundsman has an outcome hierarchy in which "5-year survival" is one "measure of overall survival."

If one could reason meaningfully on the basis of statistical grounds alone, almost all of the study's information could be captured by knowing the type of patients, the sample size, the two interventions, and the outcomes. As discussed earlier in this chapter, however, these studies cannot be used productively in clinical reasoning without expert clinical interpretation. Roundsman would provide little of value if it offered merely the statistical skeleton. Consequently, each comparison also possesses "distance metric knowledge," which is used to evaluate the clinical relevance of the statistical results to a particular patient and treatment, as described in more detail below.

In its operation, Roundsman selects certain comparisons (which are data structures located inside studies), each of which is augmented by its own dynamically assessed *distance metric*.[8] This metric consists of a set of "distances" assessing how well the comparison applies to the patient and the proposed plan. These distances include population mismatches, intervention mismatches, and methodologic weaknesses. Two examples of metric components are shown:

Long accrual period with
   se change   = increase-small
   dp change   = none
   specifics   = "patient entry lasted from 1939 to 1972"

Better prognostic stratum
   dp change   = away from zero small
   specifics   = "The study used a pooled clinical stage I and II—so that's a slightly better prognostic group than your patient."

The labels "dp change" and "se change" are slot titles referring to effects of that metric component on the difference between proportions (dp) of intervention A and intervention B, and the standard error (se) of that difference.

Components of this distance metric are used by Roundsman to analyze the clinical and statistical relevance of a particular comparison to the problem at hand. For example, in order to generate the prose output shown in the examples, the metric components were first divided (dynamically) according to whether they were (1) mismatches with the particular patient and treatment proposal or (2) methodologic issues. Within the first group, components were further divided into three subgroups: good matches, mismatches that are negligible in overall impact, and mismatches that are significant. Similarly, methodologic issues were sorted into good methodology, methodologic weaknesses of negligible impact, and serious weaknesses. Roundsman then assembled a prose discussion in the context of those subdivisions.

The metric knowledge associated with a comparison consists of one or more distance estimators. Each distance estimator contains clinical heuristics and judgments collected from our oncologist domain expert. Distance estimators are capable of contributing to (and thus enlarging) the distance metric associated with a comparison. For example, the distance estimator shown below would insert a "better prognostic stratum" distance component into the distance metric if, for the proposed treatment, a study population is in a better prognostic stratum than the physician's patient.

```
Population distance estimator with
   Outcome eq classes      = (OAS)
   Intervention1 eq classes = (any)
   Intervention2 eq classes = (any)
   Study pop classes = (clinical stages I-II)
   Patient classes      = (clinical stage II)
   Bias incurred = (a better prognostic stratum with
                       dp change  = away from zero small
                       specifics   = "The study used a pooled clinical stage
                                      I and II—so that's a slightly better prog-
                                      nostic group than your patient.")
```

The distance estimator lists "equivalence classes," which are defined on the system's outcomes, interventions, population descriptions, and patient descriptions. The system has population distance estimators (to assess mismatches between a study population and a patient) and intervention distance estimators. The population distance estimator shown above is activated (1) if the outcome being discussed in a member of the "OAS" equivalence class (any "measure of overall survival"); (2) for any interventions; (3) if the study stratum being examined by Roundsman is composed of subjects who were clinical stage I or stage II; and (d) if the physician's patient is clinical stage II. The result of activating this distance estimator is insertion of a "better prognostic stratum" distance in that comparison's metric.

If Roundsman is applied to problems other than breast cancer, certain data structures must be changed (e.g., outcomes and interventions). However, much of the current implementation generalizes to clinical studies in other medical domains.

Research Contribution

The research contribution of this project can best be understood by viewing Roundsman from the perspectives of artificial intelligence, medical decision analysis, and bibliographic retrieval.

The techniques of *artificial intelligence* are being applied to an increasing variety of problems. Biomedicine and the social sciences repeatedly present problem domains for which there are no reliable causal models. In those domains, system designers might retreat to the surface-level heuristics that sufficed for first-generation expert systems. Instead, we suggest the investigation of how experts reason from the relevant bodies of experimental evidence. This evidence may well have its own structure (as is the case for clinical literature), which is tremendously useful when combined with knowledge about how to reason based on this structure. Building computer-based models of this reasoning process may yield useful decision support systems and may also help us better understand the principles of reasoning from experimental evidence in medicine and other domains.

One of the most difficult and time-consuming parts of performing medical *decision analysis* is estimating the probability of events. It is a task that requires a strong clinical background and experience reading biostatistical reports. Furthermore, this task is common to a variety of methodologic approaches, from standard decision trees to Markov processes. There has been little explicit analysis, however, of the reasoning process by which probabilities are assigned, and (to our knowledge) no attempts to model it in a computer-based advice system. The Roundsman project explores the underlying reasoning process involved in making these assessments.

Unlike many current computer-based medical advice programs, *bibliographic retrieval* systems often meet immediate enthusiasm by clinicians. In these systems full-text copies (or abstracts) of journal articles are retrieved by a keyword index, which may be organized in a disease hierarchy or according to the keyword's proximity to another key word. These journal articles have the potential to change management decisions.[13] The state of this science, however, is primitive: Matching strings of alphanumeric characters falls far short of "intelligent" information retrieval. The current Roundsman system is a step toward the development of systems that understand the structure of the literature they are searching and can make inferences about how an article might relate to the clinical problem a physician faces.

Summary

The Roundsman project contributes to the better understanding and development of fundamental models of medical decision-making. The approach differs substantially from causal modeling in that there is no desire to model human pathophysiology but, rather, to model the structure of experimental trials and their relevance to a physician's patient and treatment plan. The development of this computational model suggests a promising new direction for medical informatics; decision support systems that bring a critical analysis of the relevant literature to the physician, structured around a particular patient and treatment plan, might be a vital addition to the tools of practicing physicians. Furthermore, computational models of how physicians reason from the clinical literature may illuminate general principles of reasoning from experimental evidence, opening these principles up to further explicit analysis.

Acknowledgments. This chapter is based on the author's PhD dissertation.[8] Dr. Rennels is supported by training grant LM-07033 from the National Library of Medicine. Dr. Shortliffe is a Henry J. Kaiser Family Foundation Faculty Scholar in General Internal Medicine. Dr. Miller is supported in part by NLM grant LM-4336. Computing resources have been provided by the Biomedical Research Technology Program under grant RR-00785 and by the Hewlett-Packard Company.

References

1. Patil RS, Szolovits P, Schwartz WB: Causal understanding of patient illness in medical diagnosis. p. 893. In: Proceedings of the 7th International Joint Conferences on Artificial Intelligence, Vancouver, 1981.
2. Davis R: Diagnostic reasoning based on structure and behavior. Artif Intell 24:347, 1984.
3. Genesereth MR: The use of design descriptions in automated diagnosis. Artif Intell 24:411, 1984.
4. Long WJ, Naimi S, Criscitiello MG, Pauker SG, Szolovits P: An aid to physiological reasoning in the management of cardiovascular disease. p. 3. In: Proceedings of the IEEE Computers in Cardiology Conference. New York: IEEE, 1984.
5. Kassirer JP, Kuipers BJ, Gorry GA: Toward a theory of clinical expertise. Am J Med 73:251, 1982.
6. Elstein AS, Shulman LS, Sprafka SA: Medical Problem Solving: An Analysis of Clinical Reasoning. Cambridge: Harvard University Press, 1978.
7. Kuipers BJ, Kassirer JP: Causal reasoning in medicine: analysis of a protocol. Cognitive Sci 8:363, 1984.
8. Rennels GD: A Computational Model of Reasoning from the Clinical Literature. New York: Springer Verlag, 1987.
9. Bailar JC, Louis TA, Lavori PW, Polansky M: A classification for biomedical research reports. N Engl J Med 311:1482, 1984.
10. Miller PL: A Critiquing Approach to Expert Computer Advice: ATTENDING. London: Pitman, 1984.
11. Fisher B, Bauer M, Margolese R, et al: Five-year results of a randomized clinical trial comparing total mastectomy and segmental mastectomy with or without radiation in the treatment of breast cancer. N Engl J Med 312:665, 1985.
12. Peters MV: Wedge resection and irradiation. Ann Intern Med 200:144, 1967.
13. Scura G, Davidoff F: Case-related use of the medical literature: clinical librarian services for improving patient care. JAMA 245:50, 1981.

11
Knowledge Acquisition and Verification Tools for Medical Expert Systems

Nicolaas J.I. Mars and Perry L. Miller

Research in artificial intelligence has shown that a large amount of domain knowledge is needed to allow expert systems to solve problems in all but the most trivial domains. The process of acquiring this knowledge (knowledge acquisition, or KA) and of determining if the knowledge is consistent, complete, and correct (knowledge verification, or KV) are time-consuming tasks that at present are major obstacles to the introduction of expert systems into many domains.

Although most designers of expert systems seem to agree that KA and KV are difficult, there are few, if any, quantitative studies of the amount of work involved. Most evidence is anecdotal. For example, Davis and Buchanan[1] mentioned that assembling a knowledge base "may involve several person-years of effort." To help alleviate this bottleneck, computer programs have been developed to assist in creating and maintaining large knowledge bases. We refer to such programs as "KA and KV tools."

The KA and KV tools can be grouped into two broad categories. Tools in the first category are designed to give the user a "better view" of a knowledge base and simpler ways of making modifications. "Intelligent" editors and graphics displays fall in this class. Tools of the second category involve the incorporation of additional knowledge and additional reasoning mechanisms used to assist the creation and refinement of a knowledge base.

This chapter outlines several approaches that have been taken when developing tools to assist in KA and KV. Because of the important role of domain knowledge in KA and KV, we confine our examples to medicine. Most of the techniques, however, are applicable to domains outside medicine as well.

Adapted from Mars NJI, Miller PL: Knowledge acquisition and verification tools for medical expert systems. *Medical Decision Making* 7:6–11, 1987. Reprinted with permission.

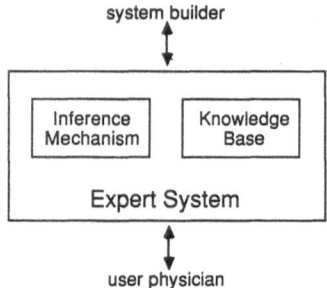

Figure 11.1. Structure of an expert system, containing a knowledge base, an inference mechanism, and two user interfaces.

Framework for Classifying KA and KV Tools

The classic structure of an expert system is shown in Figure 11.1. Here a knowledge base contains the domain knowledge that is processed by a domain-independent inference mechanism, sometimes called an "inference engine." Usually, two distinct user interfaces are provided. One user interface is for the person creating, inspecting, or modifying the knowledge base (e.g., the physician domain expert). The other is for the end-user of the system, e.g., the physician seeking advice.

To assist in the KA and KV process, additional knowledge can be brought to bear. This knowledge may, in turn, require an additional inference mechanism, as shown in Figure 11.2. As discussed later, this added knowledge base can be considered in some sense a parallel model of the domain.

For KA, the parallel model structures the process of incorporating new knowledge into the system. For KV, the parallel model provides a structure against which the system's existing knowledge base can be compared. The parallel model allows the system to interact with its knowledge base in a more intelligent and sophisticated way. Without such a parallel model of domain knowledge, a system can check its knowledge base only for overt inconsistencies, e.g., conflicts or redundancies.

Sources of Parallel Models of Domain Knowledge

There are several types of parallel model of domain knowledge that have been used to structure KA and KV. One useful classification is based on the source of the knowledge in the parallel model. Three approaches have been described.

1. Construction by the system itself by inspecting its original knowledge base
2. Construction by a (human) expert

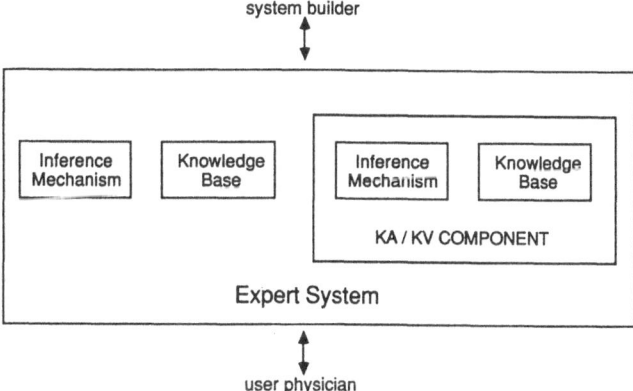

Figure 11.2. Addition of a knowledge base (a "parallel model" of the domain) and of an inference mechanism can be used to facilitate the KA and KV process.

3. Construction by the system itself from other information sources, such as experimental data gathered from the domain

Hypotheses About the Domain Inferred by the System Itself. One approach is to have the system itself infer a "parallel model" of the domain by inspecting its knowledge base. Here the system looks for patterns in its knowledge base from which it hypothesizes "generalizations." These inferred generalizations constitute expectations as to what the knowledge base should contain and are used to drive the verification of existing knowledge, the acquisition of new knowledge, or both. Because these inferred generalizations are derived by inspecting an existing knowledge base, this approach cannot be used to create the knowledge base de novo.

An advantage of this approach is that the inferred hypotheses can, in principle, be derived automatically for any domain and therefore require no extra work on the part of the domain expert. A disadvantage is that some of the hypothesized generalizations may be erroneous and may therefore lead the system to suggest modifications to its knowledge that are clearly nonsensical to someone familiar with the domain. This approach is seen in the Teiresias system, discussed later in the chapter.

Domain-Specific Model Explicitly Defined by the Domain Expert. An alternative approach is for the domain expert to outline explicitly a parallel model of certain aspects of the domain. This approach has the disadvantage that it places further demands on the domain expert beyond specifying the system's knowledge base itself. On the other hand, if the parallel model allows the knowledge base to be built and tested more efficiently, or if the parallel model is applicable to a variety of domains, these savings may more than compensate for the extra time spent creating the model.

An advantage of this approach is that the parallel model is explicitly defined by the domain expert. As a result, the model should not contain the type of overtly nonsensical errors that are possible when the model is inferred automatically. This approach is seen in the OPAL and HYDRA systems, discussed later in the chapter.

Using Experimental Data as a Model to Drive KA/KV. A third approach is to allow experimental data (e.g., test cases with known diagnoses gathered from the domain) to serve as a parallel model of the domain. Compared with the two previously described approaches, this approach has the dual advantages that (1) the domain expert need specify only the knowledge base itself, and (2) the KA/KV process is nevertheless driven by data that specifically reflect the character of the domain. This approach is taken in the SEEK system, discussed later in the chapter.

Summary. A variety of sources of parallel domain models can be used. None of the approaches is necessarily superior. Different approaches are more or less feasible and more or less successful, depending on the clinical domain and the expert system design.

Types of Knowledge in the Parallel Model

The knowledge embodied in the parallel model can be of various types. The following types have been identified in the cases to be described.

1. Knowledge about a specific domain (e.g., about the work-up of a particular medical problem)
2. Knowledge about a class of domains (e.g., about the process of medical work-up in general)
3. Knowledge about the knowledge representation formalism used, e.g., about the structure of production rules
4. Knowledge about the reasoning mechanism used

Tools That Allow Inspection of a Knowledge Base

The previous section outlined three approaches that allow the computer to assist actively in the KA/KV process, attempting to identify potential problems. A different approach is to develop tools that let the system designers inspect a knowledge base easily, perhaps using graphic techniques. Such "knowledge inspection" tools may display selected portions of the knowledge base and may even display dynamically the system's reasoning process. Using these tools the system designer performs the cognitive analysis of the knowledge displayed, e.g., by looking for potential problems. The computer facilitates this task.

Knowledge inspection tools are in a sense less ambitious than tools that interact more intelligently with a knowledge base. In part for this reason, however, knowledge inspection tools may well prove more easily implemented. As a result, such tools represent a viable approach to the KA/KV problem that may provide considerable power and flexibility to a system designer.

The expert systems described in the remainder of this chapter illustrate different parallel models, different inference mechanisms used to process those models, and different knowledge inspection tools.

Existing Tools for Knowledge Acquisition and Verification

This section describes a number of KA and KV tools that have been implemented, grouped according to the expert systems for which they were developed. Specifically, KA and KV tools are discussed for (1) MYCIN and its derivatives; (2) ONCOCIN; (3) EXPERT; and (4) other systems.

KA and KV Tools for MYCIN and Its Derivatives

MYCIN, developed at Stanford, is an expert system designed to help in the diagnosis and treatment of infectious diseases. The representation of medical knowledge using production rules, pioneered in the MYCIN system, has spawned the development of a variety of other systems and of several KA and KV tools.[2,3]

MYCIN contains several features designed to facilitate the task of the knowledge engineer.[3,4] (1) Domain knowledge, in the form of "if–then" production rules in LISP, can be entered interactively. (2) During a consultation, explanation of the system's conclusions are available, providing a trace-back of the chain of reasoning in pseudo-English. (3) A batch facility is available to allow analysis of a number of test cases (with known correct outcome) in order to study the effect of changes to the knowledge based on the system's performance. (4) The system keeps statistics as to how frequently each rule was used and its results. None of these facilities involves the use of a parallel domain model.

Despite the availability of these facilities in MYCIN, the creation of knowledge bases proved sufficiently complex and time-consuming to stimulate the development of a more sophisticated KA component, Teiresias.[1,5] Teiresias was designed explicitly to ease the knowledge engineer's task in several ways. In addition to allowing production rules to be phrased in (quasi) English, Teiresias introduced the concept of "rule models." Given a collection of rules in the knowledge base, Teiresias attempts to categorize them into classes based on their structural similarity. Thus rules leading to the same conclusions are grouped together. If at a later stage a new rule is entered with the same conclusion, Teiresias can then prompt the knowledge engineer for all predicates in the corresponding rule model to make sure that a necessary rule component was not omitted inadvertently. The final decision to accept or reject these suggestions remains with the knowledge engineer.

To show more concretely how Teiresias helps the knowledge engineer, a fragment of an interaction between a human user and Teiresias is shown below. This fragment is part of a long interaction during the debugging phase of the knowledge base. The user has indicated to the program that, for the test case under consideration, the program should have reached the conclusion that "Organism-1" (a bacterium the system is trying to recognize) may belong to the category Enterobacteriaceae.

In the transcript that follows,[2] Teiresias discusses with the user what might have gone wrong and how any problems in its knowledge base might be fixed. The user's replies are capitalized.

There were no rules successfully invoked in the attempt to deduce that the category of Organism-1 is Enterobacteriaceae.

The following (potentially applicable) rules were not executed because the starred [**] clause failed:

Rule 116
IF: 1. The identity of Organism-1 is not known
      2. The gram stain of Organism-1 is not known
           3. The morphology of Organism-1 is not known
           4. The site of Culture-1 is CSF
           5. The infection is meningitis
           6. The age (in years) of the patient is less than or equal to .17
THEN: There is weakly suggestive evidence (.3) that the category of Organism-1 is Enterobacteriaceae.

Rule 050
IF: 1. The morphology of Organism-1 is rod
           2. The gram stain of Organism-1 is gramneg
           3. The aerobicity of Organism-1 is facultative
      4. The infection with Organism-1 was acquired while the patient was hospitalized
THEN: There is evidence that the category of Organism-1 is Enterobacteriaceae.

Are all these rules correct?
+ +** YES
Should any of them have been successfully invoked?
+ +** NO
Is there a rule missing?
+ +** YES
OK, then I need a rule that would allow me to deduce that the category of Organism-1 is Enterobacteriaceae. Would you like to give me such a rule now?
+** YES

. . . .

In this example transcript, Teiresias first asks the user if the failure to correctly classify Organism-1 could be due to a mistake in one of the existing rules. When it was established that this situation was not the case, it suggested adding a rule to cover the missing case.

In a later stage of the interaction, Teiresias uses one of its inferred rule models to identify potentially missing parts of rules.

I hate to criticize, Dr. User, but did you know that most rules about what the category of an organism might be, that mention—
    The site of a culture
    The infection
Also mention—
    [A]—the portal of entry of an organism
Shall I try to write a clause to account for [A]?
+ +** YES
How about—
    [A] The portal of entry of the organism is GI
OK?
+ +** YES

The rule models are, in Davis' terminology, an example of "meta-knowledge," i.e., knowledge about knowledge. In Teiresias' case, this meta-knowledge is not accessible directly to the knowledge engineer but is used by Teiresias to drive the suggestions-prompting.

A further development, EMYCIN (essential MYCIN), contains many of the features of Teiresias and the inference mechanism of MYCIN, as well as a number of new features.[6] A more fundamental contribution are EMYCIN's facilities for performing a limited syntactic and semantic check of the knowledge base. Each newly entered rule is checked against all existing rules for *subsumption* (the rule's conclusion can be drawn from an older rule with a weaker premise) and *contradiction* (the new rule reaches a different conclusion than an older rule for the same premise). As in the case of Teiresias, the meta-knowledge that controls this analysis is not accessible to the knowledge engineer but is built into the system's code.

Two features, already present in rudimentary form in MYCIN, are much improved and expanded in EMYCIN. The first is the facility for batch analysis of a collection of test cases with known correct diagnosis. Here, in the case of incorrect diagnoses, EMYCIN adds elaborate explanations of why it reached its diagnosis and why it did not reach the diagnosis given the correct one. EMYCIN also offers a limited facility for pointing out potential erroneous interactions among rules.

Another of MYCIN's derivatives is the NEOMYCIN/HERACLES system. NEOMYCIN is an expert system specifically designed for use as a teaching system; HERACLES is its empty shell. A graphic interface for a knowledge engineer using HERACLES has been implemented in the Guidon/Watch system.[7] This interface includes a dynamic display of the reasoning process, a facility that is said to be useful to the knowledge engineer for debugging the knowledge base, as well as to the user, to better understand how a conclusion is drawn.

KA and KV Tools for the ONCOCIN System

ONCOCIN is an expert system designed to assist clinical oncologists in the management of cancer patients according to experimental treatment protocols.[8,9] ONCOCIN uses a production-rule formalism to encode knowledge from protocols. However, in contrast to MYCIN, where rules conclude with different levels of certainty, no concept of uncertainty is used. An important innovation is that all rules have an explicitly specified context in which they are applicable.

ONCOCIN contains a built-in tool to assist in the KA and KV process, the "ONCOCIN rule-checking program."[10] This rule-checker collects all rules that conclude about the same parameter and are applicable in the same context. All rules in such a collection are mutually checked for subsumption, contradiction, and incompleteness. This checking is based on the syntax of the rules only; no parallel model is available. Thus parameter value combinations that do not arise in practice owing to their semantics may give rise to warnings by the rule-checker. For this reason, the rule-checker shows all warnings to the knowledge engineer for arbitration. The designers of the rule-checker acknowledge the desirability for semantic information (i.e., fuller domain knowledge) to eliminate some of the spurious warnings.[10]

In addition to the rule-checker program, the ONCOCIN group has developed a sophisticated graphic interface between the domain expert and the ONCOCIN system, called OPAL. By requiring the domain expert to "fill in the blanks" methodically, OPAL ensures that the resulting knowledge base is complete and free of inconsistencies. Knowledge about the structure of oncology protocols forms the additional domain knowledge in OPAL. This knowledge is built into the code of the system.[11,12] Interestingly, the designers of OPAL noted that the checks inherent in the use of OPAL have uncovered several incomplete or ambiguous protocols.[12]

KA and KV Tools for the EXPERT System

The EXPERT expert system shell was derived from the expert system CASNET in much the same fashion as EMYCIN was derived from MYCIN.[13,14] SEEK[15] is a KV tool designed to help refine diagnostic knowledge bases for EXPERT. This tool starts with an initial version of the knowledge base, hand-crafted by a knowledge engineer and expressed in EXPERT's production rules. This knowledge base is assumed to be generally correct but requiring refinement. SEEK helps in this refining process.

SEEK uses as additional knowledge to guide KV a set of test cases with known (correct) conclusions. Using these test cases as a basis for its analysis, SEEK generates suggestions for possible refinements in the knowledge base. The experiments are either modest generalizations or modest specializations of the rules. The particular form of production rules used in EXPERT helps when constructing these modifications. The logic that generates the proposed experimental changes in the rules is embedded in a set of heuristic rules, which comprise another example of additional knowledge. These heuristics are domain-independent, whereas the test cases are, of course, domain-specific.

To illustrate SEEK's behavior requires some familiarity with the particular form of knowledge in EXPERT, specifically the use made in EXPERT of criteria tables. Criteria tables consist of two parts: (1) a list of major and minor observations that are significant for reaching the diagnosis; (2) a set of diagnostic rules for reaching the diagnosis.

To give a concrete example,[15] the following lists show observations for mixed connective tissue disease.

> *Major criteria*
> 1. Swollen hands
> 2. Sclerodactyly
> 3. Raynaud's phenomenon
> 4. Myositis, severe
> 5. CO diff. capacity, normally <70

> *Minor criteria*
> 1. Myositis, mild
> 2. Anemia
> 3. Pericarditis
> 4. Arthritis (≤ 6 weeks)
> 5. Pleuritis
> 6. Alopecia

The diagnostic rules for this diagnosis can be represented in tabular form (Table 11.1). Table 11.1 says, for example, that one can draw a probable diagnosis of mixed connective tissue disease if two observations from the "major criteria" list and two observations from the "minor criteria" list are present and if, additionally, the test for RNP antibody is positive.

When using SEEK, the knowledge engineer analyzes a number of test cases with a known correct diagnosis. If test cases are incorrectly classified by EXPERT, SEEK is able to suggest modifications to the criteria tables being used. For instance, if a rule incorrectly failed to diagnose a case, SEEK can suggest "generalization" experiments: Lower the number of majors or minors required, or remove requirements or exclusions. Conversely, if EXPERT reaches an erroneous diagnosis, SEEK can suggest

Table 11.1. Rules for Diagnosis

	Definite Diagnosis (4 majors)	Probable Diagnosis (2 majors, 2 minors)	Possible Diagnosis (3 majors)
Required	Positive RNP antibody	Positive RNP antibody	None
Exclusion	Positive SM antibody	None	None

"specializing" the rules for making this diagnosis, e.g., by increasing the number of majors or minors required or by adding to the list of requirements or to the list of exclusions. SEEK also can help estimate the diagnostic accuracy if the suggested changes are made. The knowledge engineer then makes the final decision to accept or reject suggested modifications.

Other Systems

An approach somewhat akin to SEEK is seen in the RX system.[16] Unlike SEEK, however, the RX system is meant to create knowledge de novo by statistical analysis of a clinical data base. Also, the RX system is not meant to be the KA component of a specific expert system but is designed to derive new medical knowledge that can be used for various purposes.

The RX system contains a hypothesis generator, a statistical test generator, and a statistical package, as well as a data base of (preclassified) cases. RX generates hypotheses (in the form of production rules) about relations between clinical parameters seen in the data base. It then generates a strategy to test these hypotheses against the observations in the data base and carries out the test strategy using its statistical package. The additional knowledge used in RX's analysis is the "scientific methodology" knowledge needed to generate and assess the hypotheses.

The RX system can be seen to be an interesting example of a potential KA and KV tool in that it aims almost to replace the domain expert and the knowledge engineer. RX is not the only example of inductive learning algorithms for KA,[17,18] it is the best known example of the inductive learning approach in a medical domain.

The Hydra system is a KA tool developed in conjunction with the Attending series of expert critiquing programs.[19] When using Hydra, a knowledge engineer constructs an augmented transition network (ATN), which represents the preferred sequence of diagnostic tests in a specific domain of work-up. Hydra analyzes this ATN, checks its consistency, and generates a set of conditions and combinations of conditions to which the critiquing system may need to react when critiquing medical work-up in that domain. The domain expert then specifies English prose comments that allow the critiquing program to react appropriately to these conditions.

A straightforward implementation of this approach, however, could generate an unwieldy number of such conditions requiring comments. To prevent it from happening, Hydra allows further domain-specific knowledge in the form of "constraints."

Conclusions

The creation and maintenance of knowledge bases can be considerably facilitated by the use of computer-based tools for knowledge acquisition and verification. A number of such tools have been described in the literature. Such tools either offer their user a better interface to view the knowledge base, or they bring additional knowledge to bear in the KA and KV process (or both).

Acknowledgments. N.J.I. Mars is supported by a Constantijn en Christiaan Huygens Fellowship from The Netherlands Organization for the Advancement of Pure Research (Z.W.O.), grant CCH 62-231. P.L. Miller is supported in part by NIH grant R01 LM04336 from the National Library of Medicine.

References

1. Davis R, Buchanan BG: Meta-level knowledge: overview and applications. p. 920. In: Proceedings of the Fifth International Joint Conference on Artificial Intelligence, 1975.
2. Buchanan BG, Shortliffe EH (eds): Rule-Based Expert Systems. Reading, MA: Addison-Wesley, 1984.
3. Shortliffe EH: Computer-Based Medical Consultations: MYCIN. New York: American Elsevier, 1976.
4. Shortliffe EH: MYCIN: A Rule-Based Computer Program for Advising Physicians Regarding Antimicrobial Therapy Selection. PhD thesis, Stanford University, 1974.
5. Davis R: Interactive transfer of expertise: acquisition of new inference rules. Artif Intell 12:121, 1979.
6. Van Melle W: A Domain-Independent System that Aids in Constructing Knowledge-Based Consultation Programs. PhD thesis, Computer Science Department, Stanford University, 1980.
7. Richer MH, Clancey WJ: Guidon-Watch: A Graphic Interface for Viewing a Knowledge-Based System. Report KSL-85-20. Stanford: Knowledge Systems Laboratory, Department of Computer Science, Stanford University, 1985.
8. Fagan L: New directions for expert systems: examples from the ONCOCIN project. p. 183. In: Proceedings of the Annual Conference of the American Association of Medical Systems and Informatics, 1984.

9. Shortliffe EH, Scott AC, Bischoff MB, Campbell AB, van Melle W, Jacobs CD: An expert system for oncology protocol management. p. 653. In Buchanan BG, Shortliffe EH (eds): Rule-Based Expert Systems. Reading, MA: Addison-Wesley, 1984.

10. Suwa M, Scott AC, Shortliffe EH: An approach to verifying completeness and consistency in a rule-based expert system. AI Magazine 2:16, 1982.

11. Musen MA, Fagan LM, Shortliffe EH: Graphical Specification of Procedural Knowledge for an Expert System. Memo KSL-85-53. Knowledge Systems Laboratory, Stanford University, 1985.

12. Musen MA, Rohn JA, Fagan LM, Shortliffe EH: Knowledge engineering for a clinical trial advice system: uncovering errors in protocol specification. p. 24. In: Proceedings of the Annual Conference of the American Association of Medical Systems and Informatics, 1986.

13. Weiss S, Kulikowski C, Safir A: Glaucoma consultation by computer. Comput Biol Med 1:25, 1978.

14. Weiss S, Kulikowski C: EXPERT: A System for Developing Consultation Models. Technical Report CBM-TR-97. New Brunswick, NJ: Rutgers University, 1979.

15. Politakis PG: Empirical Analysis for Expert Systems. Boston: Pitman, 1985.

16. Blum RL: Discovery and representation of causal relationships from a large time-oriented clinical data base: the RX project. Comput Biomed Res 15:164, 1982.

17. Bratko I, Mozetic I, Lavarac N: Automatic synthesis and compression of cardiological knowledge. In Hayes J, Michie D, Richards J (eds): Machine Intelligence. Vol. 11. Oxford: Oxford University Press, 1986.

18. Fu LM, Buchanan BG: Learning intermediate concepts in constructing a hierarchical knowledge base. p. 659. In: Proceedings of the Tenth International Joint Conference on Artificial Intelligence, 1985.

19. Miller PL, Blumenfrucht SJ, Rose JR, Rothschild M, Weltin G, Swett HA, Mars NJI: HYDRA: a knowledge acquisition tool for expert systems which critique medical workup. Med Decis Making 7:12, 1987.

12
Empirical Analysis and Refinement of Expert System Knowledge Bases

Sholom M. Weiss, Peter Politakis, and
Allen Ginsberg

Based on encouraging results in well circumscribed applications, re-searchers often propose ambitious projects to build expert systems for highly complex tasks, requiring many thousands of reasoning rules. The paradigm for designing these systems runs mainly along the lines of current expert system conventions: Knowledge engineers construct knowledge bases based on information gleaned from experts and other sources of information. In the larger, more complex applications, we can expect to have many knowledge engineers constructing a single knowledge base from multiple sources of information, with the involvement of numerous experts.

One of the major problems with such a system is to ensure expert per-formance over a sufficiently large variety of testing situations. This goal can be systematically achieved only by methods of empirical knowledge base testing and refinement.

Even when knowledge in an application is encoded in simple production rules and performance is relatively well understood, there are the major classic problems in expert systems development that pose serious obstacles in creating a complex system:

1. Knowledge acquisition.
2. Knowledge base maintenance, e.g., addition of new rules to a mature knowledge base. We can expect most knowledge bases, even well per-forming ones, to continue to undergo changes over time.
3. Knowledge base verification.

Our goal is to integrate performance information into the design of an expert model and to automatically provide advice about rule refinement. We have developed a system called SEEK[1] to generate advice in the form of suggestions for possible experiments in generalizing or specializing rules in an expert model. Case experience, stored cases with known conclusions, is used to interactively guide the expert when refining the rules of a model.

SEEK looks for regularities about the performance of the rules in mis-diagnosed cases as a basis for suggesting changes to the rules. SEEK is a system that gives interactive advice about rule refinement during the design of an expert system. The advice takes the form of suggestions for possible experiments in generalizing or specializing rules in a model of reasoning rules cited by the expert. Case experience, in the form of stored cases with known conclusions, is used to interactively guide the expert who is refining the rules of a model. This approach is most effective when the model of the expert's knowledge is relatively accurate and small changes in the model may improve performance. The system is interactive; we rely on the expert to focus the system on those experiments that appear to be most consistent with his or her domain knowledge. Examples are given from an expert consultation system being developed for diagnosing rheumatic diseases.

The SEEK system is novel in its ability to work on large-scale models with large numbers of cases and to give intelligent advice on how to en-hance the performance of an expert model. A major objective of our cur-rent research is to determine how SEEK can be extended to work with a richer class of models, e.g., a less rigid set of production rules. With the *empirical refinement approach,* we are proposing an effective solution to many of these problems for situations where examples of solved prob-lem-cases are available for testing a system. We have considerable ex-perience in applying such an approach to diagnostic classification problems formulated in a well constrained descriptive language (XP/EXPERT[2]). Because it can be expected that most practical large-scale expert system knowledge bases in the foreseeable future will be constructed using the *knowledge engineering rule* paradigm, with formal proofs of correctness being in the distant future, we are developing a more general set of prin-ciples for empirical knowledge base refinement using less restrictive se-mantics than we have in the past and exploring the extension of these methods beyond pure classification problems.

Empirical Analysis of Knowledge Base Performance

To carry out an effective empirical analysis, an additional source of in-formation is needed beyond the knowledge base supplied by the experts. This source is a collection of cases of solved examples—cases where the conclusions are known. In the best situation, these cases cover the spec-trum of possible conclusions and solution paths in a representative manner, and the cases have been independently sampled from a set not used in developing the system.

It is important to keep in perspective the role that these cases play in the development of a knowledge base. For complex knowledge bases, it is impossible to guarantee complete statistical coverage of the possible case types or solutions, so the expert-derived knowledge base is the acknowledged primary source of information for decision-making. The cases, although important, are supplementary, to be used more for purposes of quality control and consistency checking. Our expectation is that the knowledge base will be used to match the conclusions that are stored for the cases, but we hardly expect the stored cases to cover the wide spectrum of possibilities that the knowledge base must be prepared to cover. There are many analogies in real-world situations to having independent sources of decisions. For example, a well known technique for designing real-time software is to have two independent teams produce programs to perform the same task. When the programs produce different results, it is known that a serious problem has occurred.

Because these two sources of decision are not equivalent, we view them somewhat differently. For the cases stored, we accept that the stored conclusions are correct. (There are situations where this assumption may be relaxed.) We assume, however, that the knowledge base is mostly correct, and that if we detect inconsistencies with the stored cases we will only be willing to make limited adjustments to the knowledge base. It is these limited modifications that we describe as *refinements*.

SEEK generates advice in the form of suggestions for experiments for the generalization and specialization of production rules in an expert knowledge base. SEEK was the first system to integrate large-scale performance information into all phases of knowledge base development and to provide automatic information about rule refinement. The empirical analysis it performs involves gathering statistics concerning rule behavior with respect to the data base of cases. Suggestions for rule refinements are generated by the application of refinement heuristics that relate the statistical behavior and structural properties of rules to classes of rule refinements. Figure 12.1 illustrates the process of generating experiments for a knowledge base. The details of SEEK have been reported elsewhere.[1]

Here we first briefly review some of the basic principles of knowledge base refinement. In these examples we use a stylized form of decision representation consisting of two parts: (1) major and minor observations that are significant for reaching the diagnosis; and (2) a set of diagnostic production rules for reaching the diagnosis.

Uncertainty is described using three levels of confidence: *possible, probable,* or *definite.* A diagnostic rule is a conjunction of three components: specific numbers of majors or minor observations, requirements, and exclusions. As an example, the rule for concluding definite mixed connective tissue disease can be stated as follows: If the patient has four or more major observations for mixed connective tissue disease, the requirement RNP antibody is true, and the exclusion SM antibody is false, it is then concluded that definite mixed connective tissue disease is present.

The following sections focus on tools for model refinement that aid in identifying two classes of change that can be made to the rules: gener-

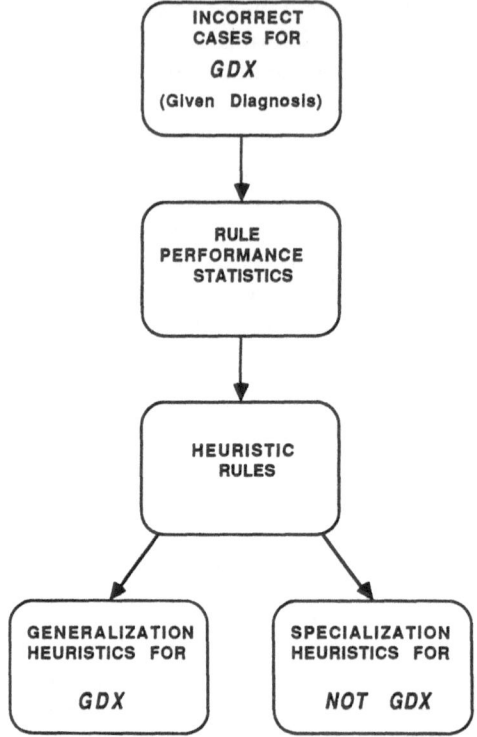

Figure 12.1. Overview of experiment generation.

alizations or specializations. *Generalizations* are changes to weaken a rule (R) that results in a different rule (R_g), where R_g logically includes R. For example, it can be accomplished by dropping a requirement or decreasing the number of major and minor findings for a rule. *Specializations* are changes to strengthen a rule (R) that results in a different rule (R_s), where R_s is logically included by R, e.g., increasing the number of major and minor findings in a rule.

Performance Summary for the Model

The performance summary is organized according to final conclusions and shows the number of cases in which the model's conclusion matches the expert's conclusion. In Table 12.1 the column labeled False Positives shows the number of cases in which the indicated conclusion was reached by the model but did not match the stored expert's conclusion. The summary of performance for mixed connective tissue disease indicates that 9 of 33 cases were correctly diagnosed. Furthermore, there are no cases that were misdiagnosed by the model as mixed connective tissue disease.

Table 12.1. Summary of Performance

Disease	True Positive		False Positive
Mixed connective tissue disease	9/33	(27%)	0
Rheumatoid arthritis	42/42	(100%)	9
Systemic lupus erythematosus	12/18	(67%)	4
Progressive systemic sclerosis	22/23	(96%)	5
Polymyositis	4/5	(80%)	1
Total	89/121	(74%)	

The rules that conclude rheumatoid arthritis perform well for the stored rheumatoid arthritis cases, but they also appear to be candidates for specialization because of the nine false positives.

Analysis of the Model Based on Case Experience

The first step for the analysis of a model based on case experience is to specify a final diagnosis for which rules are to be analyzed. In this manner, the model designer focuses the analysis on a subset of the rules in the model. The analysis is usually done after performance results for all diagnoses have been obtained. SEEK assists the model designer in the analysis of a subset of the rules that are relevant to the misdiagnosed cases. An important design consideration for SEEK is to provide the model designer with a flexible means to perform experiments when refining the rules. Advice can be given that helps to determine the specific experiments for rule refinement. Heuristic procedures are needed to select experiments from the many possibilities. For example, SEEK uses a heuristic procedure to determine which rules for the expert's conclusion are closest to being satisfied in a misdiagnosed case. It looks for a partially satisfied rule in a case for which the following conditions hold:

1. The rule concludes at a minimum confidence level that is greater than the certainty value for the model's conclusion.
2. The rule contains the maximum number of satisfied components for all rules concluding at that confidence level.

A rule satisfying these conditions is marked for generalization (weakening), so that it may be invoked more frequently. The rule used to reach the model's conclusion is marked for specialization (strengthening), so it may be invoked less frequently.

The scheme for the analysis of the cases focuses on a subset of the rules by gathering empirical information suggesting the generalization and specialization of rules in the set. It can be viewed as a learning system that limits changes to refinements of existing rules. In Mitchell's version space approach,[3] two sets of rules are maintained as bounds on the maximally specialized rules and the maximally generalized rules that are consistent with the training cases presented for a conclusion. A training case is prespecified as either positive (a rule must be found to cover the case) or negative (no rule should match the case). The scheme seeks to cover all positive cases while allowing no negative cases to match any of the rules. There are no certainty values assigned to the rules in the version space. Our scheme seeks to refine expert-derived rules that have been categorized by confidence levels in the model. Correct classification for all cases is not required. That is, a negative case is allowed to be covered so long as there is a rule for another conclusion that overrides the matched rule(s). A rule is marked for generalization or specialization based on the comparison of the certainty values assigned to the conclusion of the expert and the conclusion reached by the model. Finally, our scheme is interactive in nature, requiring the involvement of the model designer. It is not intended to be an autonomous learning system.

Heuristics for Suggesting Experiments

Heuristics are needed to suggest specific rule refinement experiments from the many possibilities that could be tried to correct misdiagnosed cases. Situations often arise where the empirical evidence supports both generalization and specialization of the same rule. In one misdiagnosed case, a satisfied rule could have been found to be responsible for incorrectly diagnosing the case. On the other hand, the same rule could have been unsatisfied in several other misdiagnosed cases where, if it were satisfied, the rule could have correctly diagnosed these cases. Given this situation, one would reasonably focus on ways to weaken the rule in contrast to strengthening it because the empirical evidence favors this approach. Thus a generalization experiment would be needed so the rule may be satisfied in the subset of misdiagnosed cases to which this rule should be applied. The heuristics must therefore contain information about a rule's performance in order to determine whether to weaken or strengthen a rule. Furthermore, other empirical information is needed to select a specific experiment. In the case of a generalization experiment, there must be a way to determine the specific component(s) that should be removed from the rule. It means that we need to gather statistics about a rule's performance on a data base of cases. An example of a heuristic rule for suggesting an experiment to decrease the number of majors in a rule is shown in Figure 12.2.

The generation of advice about rule refinement is a two-stage process. The first stage involves gathering statistics about rule performance as a result of analyzing all cases in the data base. The second stage is the evaluation of the heuristic rules using the statistics showing the rules' performance for the purpose of suggesting specific experiments about rule refinement. The potential loss as a result of generalizing a rule by either

IF: The number of cases suggesting generalization of the rule is greater than the number of cases suggesting specialization of the rule and
the most frequently missing component in the rule is the *MAJOR* component,

THEN: *Decrease the number of major findings in the rule.*

Figure 12.2. Example of heuristic rule for suggesting an experiment.

removing a component or increasing the confidence is the increase in the number of false positives already attributed to the rule. The exact impact of a change is ascertained by trying an experiment that conditionally incorporates a change into the model and tests the model on the data base of cases.

Generation of Model Refinement Experiments

In general, there are many possibilities that can be tried for refining the rules in a model. A heuristic rule-based scheme is used to suggest experiments. The IF part of the heuristic rule contains a conjunction of predicate clauses that looks for certain features about the performance of rules in the model, and the THEN part of the heuristic rule contains a specific rule refinement experiment. An example of a heuristic rule is shown in Figure 12.2 and was used to suggest the specific generalization experiment to decrease the number of major findings in a rule. Currently, there are about a dozen heuristic rules that are divided almost equally with respect to the types of experiments (i.e., generalizations or specializations) that may be suggested.

Evaluation of a heuristic rule begins by instantiating the clauses with the required empirical information about a specific rule in the model. The experiments suggested for the rules used in reaching the diagnosis of mixed connective tissue disease are as follows.

1. Decrease the number of majors in rule 56.
2. Delete the requirement component in rule 55.
3. Delete the requirement component in rule 54.
4. Decrease the number of minors in rule 57.
5. Delete the requirement component in rule 58.

One is not absolutely certain of a net gain in performance before an actual experiment is tried by running the entire data base of cases through the modified model. It comes about because interactions among rules cannot be practically predicted *a priori* in a large model where the number of possibilities is large.

Reviewing the Refinement Experiments

The results of a specific experiment are obtained by conditionally incorporating the revised rule(s) into the model. The updated model is then executed on the data base of cases. The results are summarized in Table 12.2, which compares the performance before and after the rule modification. On the basis of such a summary, the model designer can choose whether to accept or reject the experiment, proceed to other related experiments, or try a totally different approach.

Second Generation SEEK System

The original SEEK program was an important first step in realizing our research goal. Its success proved that case knowledge and knowledge-engineering concepts and heuristics can be integrated into a useful tool that uses empirical analysis to suggest model refinements. Our experience with SEEK has convinced us that the construction of a more powerful and flexible model refinement system using this approach is both desirable and feasible. We have already implemented a major portion of SEEK's successor, SEEK2. Below we describe what has been done, as well as our ideas for SEEK2's future development. In this section we describe how SEEK2 works, i.e., how it is used to help refine a knowledge base.

From a conceptual point of view, it is convenient to think of SEEK2 as having a basic cycle of operation, which consists of a number of phases and which is repeated until the user is satisfied with the resulting domain model. At the start of each cycle the system has a current version of the domain model and a data base of cases containing the expert's case knowledge. SEEK2 first obtains a *performance evaluation* of the current model on the data base of cases. This step is done by running the current model on each of the cases in the data base and then comparing the model's conclusion with the stored expert conclusion. The performance evaluation consists primarily of a breakdown by diagnosis of the number of cases in which the model agrees with the expert in reaching a particular diagnosis, i.e., *true positives*, and the number of cases in which the model reaches that diagnosis but the expert does not, i.e., *false positives*.

At this point the user must decide on a category of diagnosis for which

Table 12.2. Summary of Before/After Performance

Model	Before	After
MCTD	9/33 (27%)	17/33 (52%)
Others	80/88 (91%)	80/88 (91%)
Total	89/121 (74%)	97/121 (80%)

he would like to see refinements in the model in order to obtain better performance; e.g., if the domain is rheumatology, the user may decide to try to upgrade the model's performance in diagnosing rheumatoid arthritis (RA). For the sake of brevity, we call this user-specified diagnosis the GDX for the current cycle of operation, where the G stands for *given*, as the user has to give this information to the system.

The next part of the cycle involves *gathering statistical information concerning the rules of the model that conclude the GDX*. SEEK2 is equipped with a set of domain-independent statistical concepts that are useful when coming to decisions concerning the desirability of modifying the rules in the model in certain ways. One statistic of interest, for example, involves the number of times a particular rule is solely responsible for a misdiagnosed case, in the sense that if the rule had not been satisfied the model would otherwise have reached the correct conclusion; this statistic is a function of the rules in the model, and we call it SpecA(rule). Continuing with the rheumatology example, if the GDX is RA and rule r concludes RA, in the statistics-gathering phase of its cycle one of the pieces of information that SEEK2 computes is SpecA(r). For future use we mention another example of a statistic gathered in this phase, viz., the number of cases in which r has the sole responsibility for the correct diagnosis, i.e., cases in which if r had not been satisfied the model would have reached an incorrect diagnosis. In SEEK2 this concept is represented by the function called Signif(r).

The knowledge of how one should use these statistics in arriving at decisions to modify the rules of the model is embodied in SEEK2 in the form of a set of heuristic rules. Once the statistics have been collected for every rule that concludes the GDX, each of these heuristics is evaluated for every rule in turn. As an example, a simplified version of one heuristic says that if SpecA(r) is greater than Signif(r)—i.e., the satisfaction of rule r is the sole reason for the model's incorrect conclusion in more cases than it is the sole reason for the model's correct conclusion—it may be advisable to modify rule r in such a way as to make it more difficult to be satisfied. The justification for this heuristic in brief is that, other things being equal, because SpecA(r) is bigger than Signif(r) it is likely that by making it more difficult for r to be satisfied we will correct more cases in the SpecA(r) set than we will lose in the Signif(r) set; that is, the model's performance with respect to the GDX is likely to experience a net gain.

We group SEEK2's heuristics into two categories according to the general nature of the rule modifications they suggest. *Generalization heuristics* are those whose recommendations are aimed at making it more likely that the rule in question is responsible for the model's conclusion in any given case; *specialization heuristics* are those whose recommendations are aimed at making it less likely that the rule in question is responsible for the model's conclusion in any given case. Each heuristic actually recommends a specific way in which a rule may be generalized or specialized. For example, a rule can be specialized by adding a new component to it, altering one of its existing components in such a way that it is more difficult to satisfy, or lowering its confidence factor. The first two alternatives attempt to lessen the impact of a rule by making it more difficult for it to be satisfied; the last alternative makes it less likely that the rule's conclusion will be taken as the model's diagnosis even when it is satisfied. Furthermore, whenever SEEK2 suggests specializing a rule, the user has the option of asking the system to conduct further empirical analyses that will result in the recommendation of a specific component to modify in the rule.

After SEEK2 has given its advice—we think of each piece of advice as a possible experiment to improve the model—the user decides on which recommendations to incorporate in the model and changes the model accordingly. This phase marks the end of the current cycle. The cycle may now be repeated with the modified model, and this process may continue until the user is satisfied with the overall performance evaluation.

The current implementation of SEEK2 contains a number of features that mark it as a significant advance over SEEK. (1) SEEK2 works with a more general class of knowledge bases than SEEK; (2) SEEK2 has an automatic pilot capability, i.e., it can, if desired, perform all of the basic tasks involved in knowledge base refinement without human interaction; (3) a meta-language for knowledge base refinement has been specified that describes both domain-independent and domain-specific meta-knowledge about the refinement process.

Future Directions

The SEEK system is a real system that functions on real knowledge bases. It has been fully tested on one moderately sized knowledge base (several hundred rules) and has been independently used to develop and test another medical knowledge base.[4] SEEK2 has demonstrated improvements for the same knowledge base on which SEEK was originally tested.[5]

Several new directions in empirical refinement systems appear promising:

1. Generalization of problem types covered by refinement
2. Development of a knowledge base language
3. Incorporation of domain-specific heuristics
4. Exploitation of parallelism in certain refinement operations
5. Inclusion of automatic learning heuristics

Generalization of Problem Types and Knowledge Base Language

SEEK2, which has become our experimental vehicle for research, accepts a significant portion of the XP/EXPERT language.[2] It has allowed us to experiment with real world medical diagnosis knowledge bases. The language is limited to production rules applied to classification problems—a significant class of problems that characterize many expert system applications—but other problems classes may be considered as well, e.g., sequential action selection (stylized planning programs). The specification and implementation of a new meta-language that augments the production rule representation should prove valuable. Even within our current refinement framework, several useful representational structures have been deliberately excluded for the sake of simplicity, including taxonomic relations, notions of context, negative scoring confidence factors, and more complex scoring functions. As we move to include these more sophisticated representational components, interesting issues arise concerning the trade-offs between the degree of structural complexity of relations used in a knowledge base and the ability to analyze and refine the knowledge base.

A natural step is to develop a meta-language knowledge base language in such a way that not only can SEEK2's heuristics be represented but also SEEK2's statistics. The idea is to come up with a few well chosen primitive concepts that would be built into the language (e.g., the concept of a case, a conclusion) and a few well chosen ways in which these primitives could be combined to form new concepts (e.g., set formation, conjunction). This language could be used not only to define and explore the effects of modifications to SEEK2's existing statistical concepts, e.g., $SpecA(r)$, it could also be made accessible to the general user of the system, so that other statistics and heuristics could be incorporated into SEEK2.

A good start has been made in the fundamental conceptual work needed to achieve this goal. Extensive progress has been made in developing a system that accepts descriptions of statistical and heuristic concepts to be tested on case data and a SEEK2 knowledge base.[6]

Domain Specific Heuristics

The SEEK2 system has 12 powerful heuristic rules that prune its search over the knowledge base to a relatively small number of potential experiments. Our experience to date suggests that these heuristics are generally domain-independent and hold for most knowledge bases created in the target language. However, there are many problems for which domain-specific knowledge about potential refinements to the knowledge base can be helpful and can allow more circumscribed and efficient generation of refinements. A simple example is that a certain rule component X should never be modified in any rule that is activated by context Y. A different set of language constructs is needed to describe this type of knowledge, and to investigate the advantages of domain-independent versus domain-independent refinements.

Once such capabilities are developed, more complex refinements than are currently being generated by SEEK2 could be attempted on practical large-scale knowledge bases. Although one can now easily see how such experiments can be generated, the complexity of these generation procedures are enormous. With domain knowledge, the generation process can be pruned dramatically. The use of domain-specific knowledge, in the form of a deeper model of domain knowledge,[7] is the most prominent alternative to the empirical approach that we have taken in SEEK2. However, these approaches are not mutually exclusive.

Parallelism

The current SEEK2 procedure for generating refinements can be a time-consuming task. The time taken is related to many factors including the number of rules, the number of endpoints (conclusions), and the number of cases. For a large knowledge base, even with the heuristic search techniques that are used we can expect a significant amount of computer processing time to be expended. It appears, however, that the SEEK2 search problem is made to order for parallel architectures and that adaptation of the current procedures would be relatively easy. We expect to experiment with this possibility, combining this idea with an augmented language that allows the knowledge engineer to specify additional parallel efficiencies.

Evolution from Refinement to Learning

Although significant efforts have been expended on building automatic learning systems, they are rarely practical for building large-scale, sophisticated expert knowledge bases. A realistic approach is to start with an existing knowledge base and a refinement system that first suggests experiments and carries out the fine-tuning of those rules that are close to being correct. However, for parts of the knowledge base that show severe problems of performance, it would be reasonable to go beyond refinement heuristics and experiment with radical changes to the knowledge structures and rules. Having a system that combines domain-independent and domain-dependent learning and refinement heuristics allows us to investigate the gradual evolution of system capabilities so as to incorporate successive degrees of skepticism when challenging the original knowledge base. In this way we start with modest capabilities of learning from the solved case examples and gradually evolve to accepting their results in a fashion that responds intelligently to weaknesses in the structure of the original knowledge base. Having in SEEK2 a system that already accepts the specification of knowledge for real-world problems is clearly advantageous. The notion of learning can be introduced by allowing the system to not only refine rules but in some instances to add a completely new rule component or even a completely new rule. Such learning may be attempted based on case knowledge, although domain specific knowledge is of even greater importance in the learning task.

New Applications

The SEEK system has been developed using a rheumatology knowledge base and data base. We expect that the rheumatology application will continue to be enhanced and will therefore continue to be a rich source of experimental data for the SEEK system. Because the newer SEEK2 system can process a more generalized format of decision rules, the opportunity exists to test our ideas on other applications, which we expect to do in a new application of laboratory medicine. Such application will provide a unique opportunity for an expert system to modify itself based on local population statistics. The extent to which it can be accomplished successfully will be driven by the capabilities of the computer science techniques and the validity of applying these techniques to this specific laboratory medicine application.

SEEK2 is a vehicle for investigating empirical knowledge refinement, which can lead to an experimental knowledge-based system that has well defined capabilities of learning from experience. The lack of this capability is a major weakness in contemporary expert systems. We are extending the capabilities of the existing system SEEK2 to allow experimentation with various degrees of knowledge structure and different levels of domain dependence in the refinement heuristics. It should provide valuable insights into how practical knowledge refinement systems ought to be designed so as to fruitfully combine detailed tracing and justification of performance in single case analyses with large-scale, more statistical evaluation of performance over an entire knowledge base.

Acknowledgment. This work was supported in part by NIH grant P41-RR02230.

References

1. Politakis P, Weiss S: Using empirical analysis to refine expert system knowledge bases. Artif Intell 22:23, 1984.
2. Weiss S, Kulikowski C: A Practical Guide to Designing Expert Systems. Totowa, NJ: Rowman & Allanheld, 1984.
3. Mitchell T: Generalization as search. Artif Intell 18:203, 1982.
4. Vanker A, Stoecker W: An expert diagnostic program for dermatology. Comput Biol Med 17:241, 1984.
5. Ginsberg A, Weiss S, Politakis P: SEEK2: a generalized approach to automatic knowledge base refinement. p. 367. In: Proceedings of the Ninth International Joint Conference on Artificial Intelligence, Los Angeles, 1985.
6. Ginsberg A: Refinement of Expert System Knowledge Bases: A Metalinguistic Framework for Heuristic Analysis. PhD thesis, Department of Computer Science, Rutgers University, 1986.
7. Smith R, Winston H, Mitchell T, Buchanan B: Representation and use of explicit justification for knowledge base refinement. p. 673. In: Proceedings of the Ninth International Joint Conference on Artificial Intelligence, Los Angeles, 1985.

13
OPAL: Toward the Computer-Aided Design of Oncology Advice Systems

Mark A. Musen, David M. Combs,
Joan D. Walton, Edward H. Shortliffe, and
Lawrence M. Fagan

Creating the knowledge base of an expert system, as when developing any model, requires the abstraction of some reality. The important aspects of a problem area must be identified and extracted. The often difficult process of identifying, extracting, and representing those important domain aspects for use by an expert system is called *knowledge acquisition*. Successful knowledge acquisition is often considered the major obstacle in the construction of knowledge-based advice systems.[1]

Although some physicians with limited training have learned to use existing knowledge acquisition tools to construct small expert systems,[2] it is in general unrealistic to expect medical personnel to learn the computer programming skills and knowledge representation techniques required to build production-quality programs. For the development of robust expert systems, the traditional approach to knowledge acquisition still applies: Specially trained computer scientists, called *knowledge engineers*, must painstakingly interview experts in the application area and encode the experts' problem-solving knowledge for the computer. Because knowledge engineers are typically unfamiliar with the vocabulary and structure of an application area, and because the experts often have little appreciation for how their knowledge should be incorporated into the knowledge base of an expert system, knowledge acquisition is characteristically a slow, tedious, and highly iterative process.

It is possible, however, to facilitate knowledge acquisition if one can bypass the need for a knowledge engineer to mediate between the domain expert and the knowledge base. One approach is for the expert to work alone using an intelligent *knowledge-editing program*.[3] Although such computer-based tools have been developed to assist in either the early formalization of knowledge bases[4,5] or refinement of relatively mature systems,[6,7] little work has focused on expediting the development of new knowledge bases when the application area is already well conceptualized.

At Stanford we have been developing a program for knowledge ac-

© 1986 by the Institute of Electrical and Electronics Engineers, Inc. Reprinted with permission, from *Proceedings of the 10th Annual Symposium on Computer Applications in Medical Care*, Washington, D.C., October 25–26, pp. 43–52.

quisition called OPAL. OPAL allows specialists in cancer therapy to enter and review the knowledge of oncology treatment plans encoded for an expert system called ONCOCIN,[8,9] which recommends specific treatment for cancer patients. The goal in OPAL is to bypass dependence on knowledge engineers by allowing oncologists to enter knowledge directly into the computer. By modeling elements of the application area using computer graphics, OPAL attempts to create an environment that allows oncology experts, working alone, to specify new cancer treatment plans for ON-COCIN.[10,11] One can think of the approach explored in OPAL as the computer-aided design of new knowledge bases.

Cancer Therapy and ONCOCIN

Because optimal treatment for most malignancies is not known, cancer patients are often enrolled in formal experiments, or *clinical trials,* that compare the effects of alternative treatment plans for the same disease. The written descriptions of these experiments are called *protocols.* Patients are typically assigned at random to one of a protocol's alternative treatments. When sufficient numbers of patients complete therapy according to the protocol, statistical analysis of their outcomes allows determination of which of the competing treatment plans is preferable.

Oncology protocols may be complex. They typically mandate various *chemotherapies* (groups of one or more drugs given over time), radiation treatments, or surgery. An individual treatment plan may combine multiple chemotherapies (each with its own sequence of drugs) with radiotherapy or surgery. Typically, administration of the drugs in a chemotherapy is repeated several times, each referred to as a *cycle* of treatment. The repetition may be fixed beforehand (e.g., "Repeat eight times") or vary according to changes in the patient's condition (e.g., "Repeat until there is disease progression"). Oncology protocols may also dictate *concurrent* actions, as patients may undergo cycles of chemotherapy and radiation treatments simultaneously.

The drugs used to treat cancer are uniformly toxic. An important aim of cancer chemotherapy is to maximize the amount of drug given to a patient to control the tumor without causing intolerable side effects. Consequently, oncology protocols contain large numbers of detailed specifications that modify therapy based on the extent of a patient's cancer and the presence of treatment-induced toxicity.

ONCOCIN is able to recommend treatment for cancer patients because it has a large knowledge base of oncology protocols. The knowledge base can be viewed as containing two classes of knowledge: one *procedural* and one *inferential.*

The *procedural component* of the knowledge base describes the performance of sequences of actions over time. At the highest level it is used to describe the ordering, or *algorithm,* of the various chemotherapies and radiotherapies being administered to the patient. Procedural knowledge is encoded in a structure known as a *generator,* which is used by ON-COCIN to define a patient's progression between the various states in the treatment plan.[12] When making a treatment recommendation for a particular patient visit, ONCOCIN examines the generator describing the appropriate protocol to determine the type of chemotherapy or radiotherapy to be administered.

After consulting the generator for the general treatment plan, ON-COCIN uses the inferential component of the knowledge base to refine the plan. Using a hierarchy of highly structured knowledge base objects called *frames* and *if–then rules* associated with those frames,[13] ONCOCIN reasons about the precise treatment that should be given based on its knowledge of the protocol, the patient's past response to treatment,[14] and current patient data.

The current version of ONCOCIN runs on single-user professional work stations with large, bit-mapped displays and "mouse" pointing devices.[15] The program has been totally redesigned from an earlier prototype that ran on a large, time-shared computer.[8] The current knowledge base of 36 oncology protocols in the work-station version of ONCOCIN has been entered largely using OPAL, which was developed as a knowledge-entry tool for use by our collaborating oncologists. Because these physicians know little about the internal workings of ONCOCIN, OPAL hides the existence of the generators, frames, and rules. Instead, it displays oncology knowledge in a simple graphic format that is readily understood by physicians. As a result, clinical experts can rapidly enter new protocols for ONCOCIN without having to understand programming.

Entry of Procedural Knowledge

In their written descriptions of protocols, oncologists typically depict the sequence of high-level steps in a treatment plan using a flow chart, or *schema* (Fig. 13.1). OPAL provides oncologists with a visual programming language[16] that allows them to construct analogous flow charts using special graphic symbols called *icons* (Fig. 13.2).

The initial OPAL display is devoted to a large rectangular region where the user creates the visual program representing a particular protocol schema. Below this area is a palette of "reference" icons that correspond to some of the basic elements of the visual language (Fig. 13.3). The icons include basic control operators such as START (begin protocol), STOP (terminate the protocol), and DECIDE (binary branch), as well as the basic treatment modalities CHEMOTHERAPY and RADIOTHERAPY. An operator labeled WAIT can be used to designate explicit pauses in treatment.

When the user selects one of the reference icons with the mouse pointing

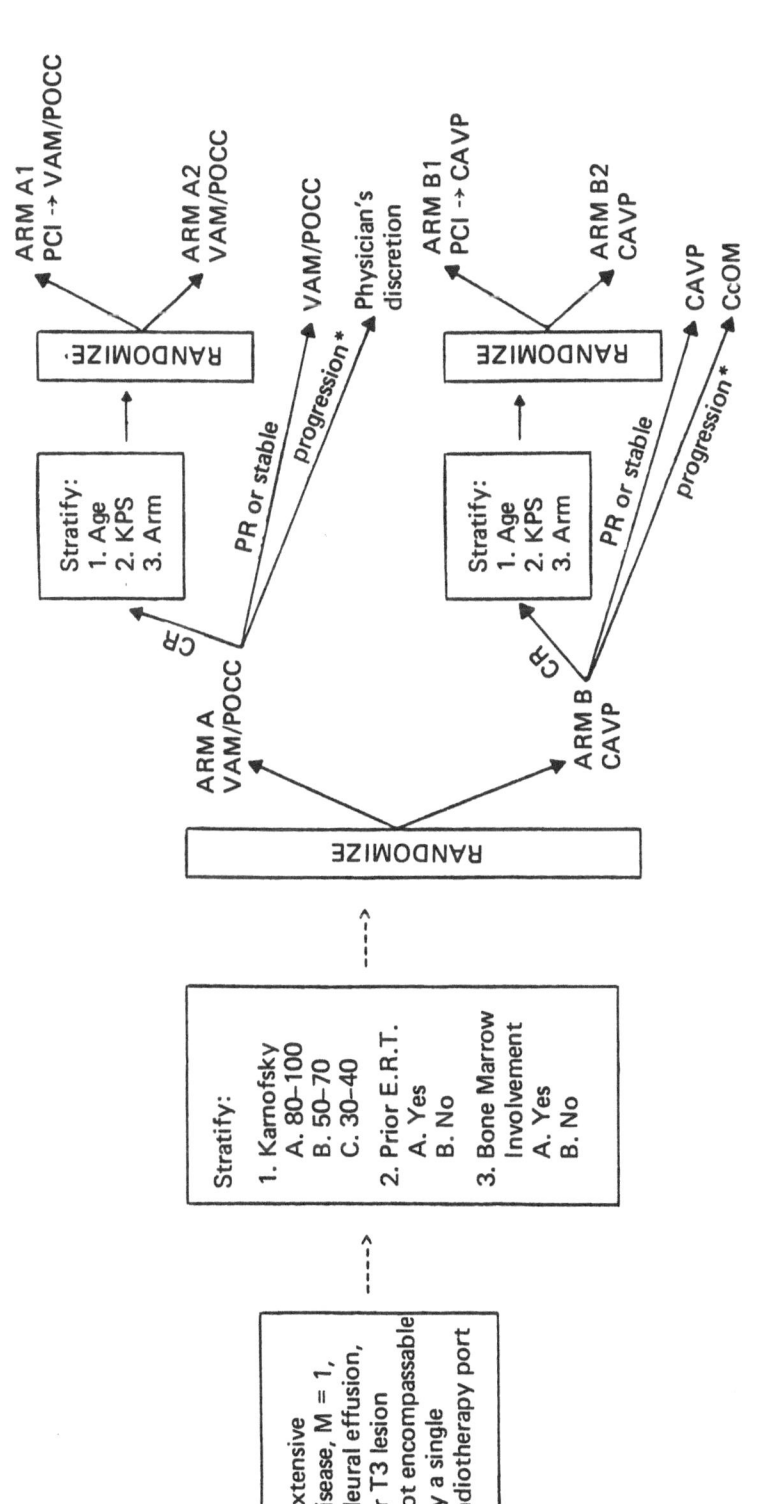

Figure 13.1. Sample protocol schema. This diagram is taken directly from Northern California Oncology Group protocol 20-83-1 for small cell lung cancer. Patients are randomly assigned to either arm A, which tests the chemotherapies VAM and POCC, or arm B, which tests the chemotherapy CAVP. Patients who have complete response (CR) to either treatment arm may be randomly assigned to receive prophylactic cranial irradiation (PCI) in addition to continued chemotherapy.

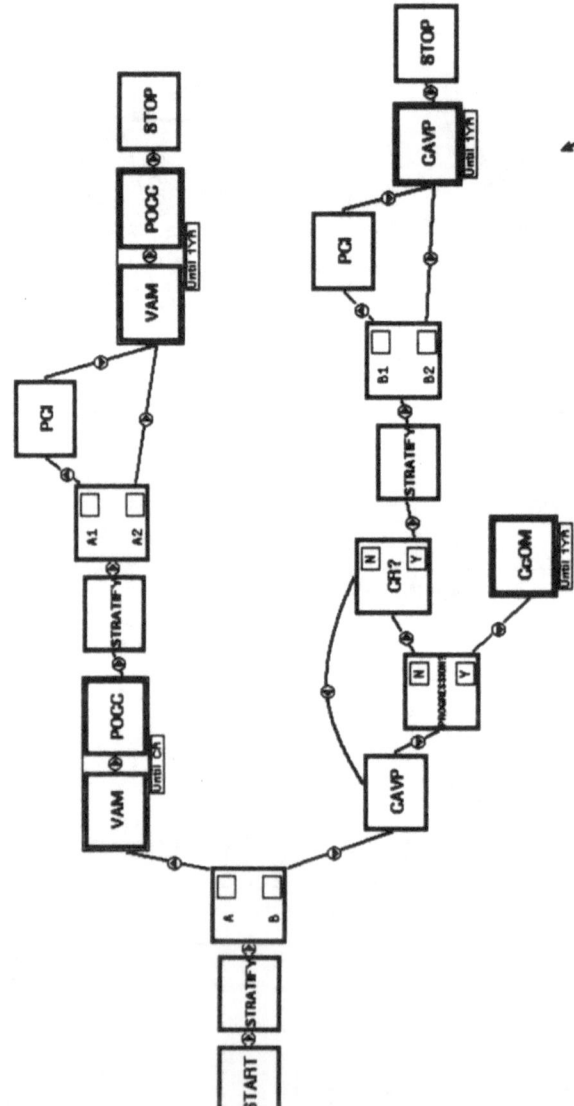

Figure 13.2. Schema for protocol entered with OPAL. This schema is a modified version of that for Northern Calfornia Oncology Group protocol 20-83-1 entered with OPAL as seen on the computer display. Note the relation of this graphic description to the flow diagram from the protocol document shown in Figure 13.1.

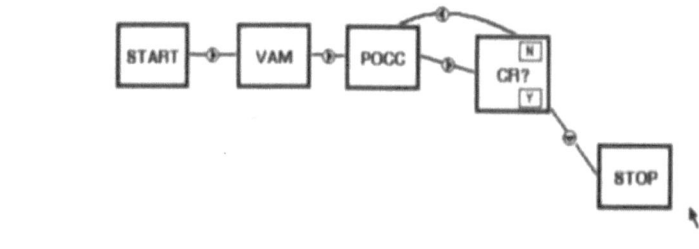

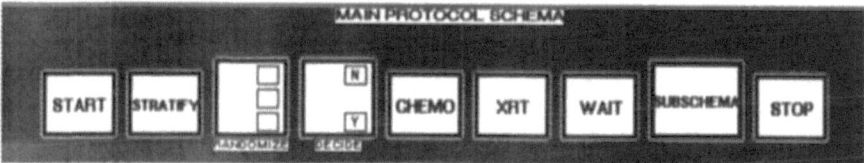

Figure 13.3. OPAL schema entry environment. Below the region where the user edits the schema is a palette of "reference" icons, used to add new nodes to the flow chart. These icons include such basic control elements as START, STOP, and DECIDE, as well as specific domain processes, e.g., chemotherapy cycles (CHEMO) and radiation treatments (XRT, for x-ray therapy). The schema that has been constructed calls for a single cycle of VAM chemotherapy to be administered, followed by cycles of POCC chemotherapy until the parameter CR (complete response) becomes true. The visual program is automatically translated by OPAL into an internal representation called a *generator*.

device, a copy of the icon appears in the main schema region. The new icon may be positioned anywhere in the region by moving the mouse. If the user adds a CHEMOTHERAPY or RADIOTHERAPY icon, the particular form of the treatment is selected from a menu that pops up after the icon is moved into place. The name chosen from the menu then appears as a label for the icon. Similarly, if the user creates a DECIDE node in the schema, a menu of ONCOCIN knowledge base *parameters* is displayed. (The values of parameters in ONCOCIN are concluded by rules and reflect such concepts as the patient's condition or stage of treatment.) The user is asked to specify the name of the parameter whose value during the ONCOCIN consultation determines the flow of control at the branch point.

The user creates a visual program for the protocol schema by adding icons to the graph, positioning them appropriately, and drawing links between them. When an icon previously added to the graph is selected with the mouse, a menu appears, allowing it to be moved elsewhere, erased from the graph, or linked to another icon. If a link between icons is selected with the mouse, the user can erase the link from the diagram or change the link's destination. OPAL thus provides a "what you see is what you get" environment for drawing out protocol schemas. Detailed protocol flow charts can be created rapidly.

Visual programming in OPAL possesses many of the same syntactic and semantic constructs ordinarily associated with textual programming languages such as PL/I or Ada. Sequential control, conditionality, iteration, concurrency, and exception handling can all be represented using a graphic notation. In addition, abstraction of complex procedures as graphic "subroutines" is possible using the SUBSCHEMA icon.[12]

After verifying that there are no syntactic errors in the design of the flow chart (e.g., missing links between icons), OPAL automatically translates the visual representation of the protocol algorithm into a generator for incorporation into the ONCOCIN knowledge base. The user never needs to be concerned with ONCOCIN's internal representation of the graphically entered knowledge.

Forms-Based Knowledge Entry

There is a second class of ONCOCIN knowledge that is not concerned with the procedural aspects of cancer protocols. Rather, it specifies how the administration of particular chemotherapies and radiotherapies should be modified based on the condition of the patient. Whereas such *inferential* knowledge is represented internally in ONCOCIN as frames and rules, OPAL permits physicians to enter this aspect of the knowledge base using graphic *forms*[17] (Fig. 13.4).

OPAL provides a convenient interface between the iconic schema-entry environment and the forms-based portion of the system. In general, physicians first use OPAL to draw out the protocol schema, as in Figure 13.2. At any time, it is possible to select one of the elements of the schema diagram with the mouse and to indicate the desire to specify "details." The schema-entry environment is then replaced with a menu of possible forms for specification of the inferential knowledge pertaining to the selected element. The user can fill out the forms and, with a simple click of the mouse button, return to the "top level" schema environment.

The forms in OPAL have been designed to be understandable to physicians. In some cases the forms actually reproduce tables customarily found in oncology protocol documents (Fig. 13.5). The content of the forms reflects a detailed model of the knowledge expected in oncology protocols.[11] The strong assumptions made by OPAL concerning the structure of the domain reduces forms-based knowledge entry to the simple process of filling in blanks from menus of possible values. For example, the form in Figure 13.4 allows the user to specify the names of the individual drugs that make up a particular chemotherapy. Pointing at one of the blanks with the mouse causes a menu of all drugs known to the system to appear. Choosing one of the drugs from the menu causes the selected drug name to replace the previous contents of the blank. (Alternatively, a drug name can be typed in from the keyboard.) When a blank requesting a

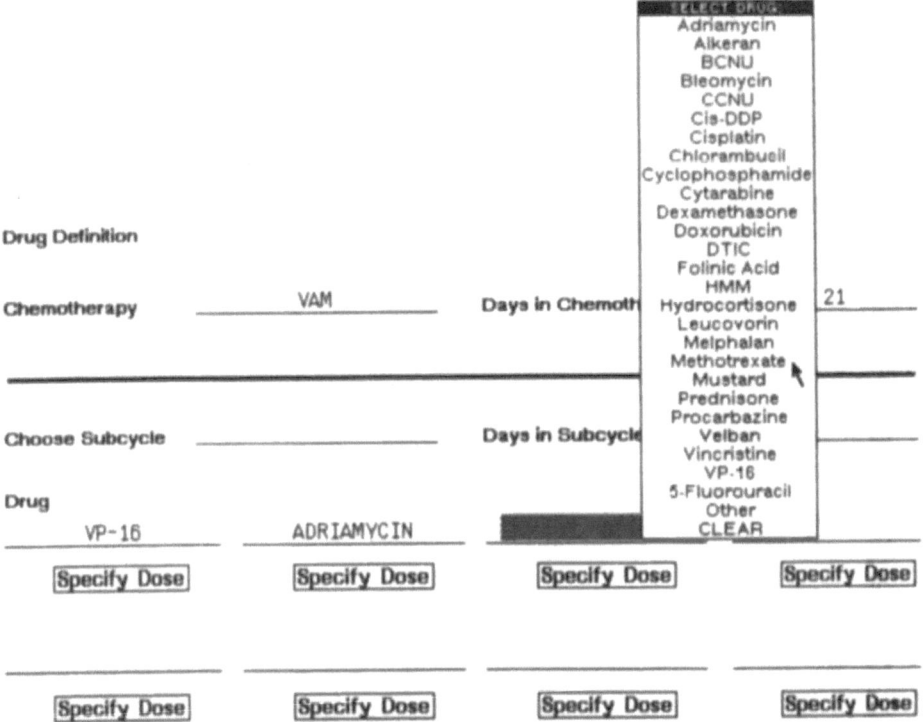

Figure 13.4. Forms-based knowledge entry. This form displays information concerning drug combinations (in this case VAM, which consists of VP-16, Adriamycin, and methotrexate). The user has already entered the names of the first two drugs in the form and is about to select the third drug from the menu. OPAL creates a separate knowledge base element called a *frame* for each drug.

drug name is filled in, knowledge stored in the internal representation of the OPAL form causes the creation of a new *frame* in the knowledge base for the indicated drug. When the user selects the box labeled *Specify Dose* beneath one of the drug names in Figure 13.4, another OPAL form is displayed in which certain properties of the designated drug can be entered. Knowing how the user invoked the new form (i.e., knowing which box in the first form was selected) allows OPAL to store the information in the appropriate frame.

OPAL may also be used to create rules in the ONCOCIN knowledge base. For instance, the form in Figure 13.6 allows the user to denote protocol modifications that are based on laboratory tests. In this example, the expert has indicated that when a patient's serum creatinine is greater than 1.5 mg/dl, the drug methotrexate should be withheld from VAM chemotherapy. The values entered by the physician correspond to a pro-

PERCENT OF CALCULATED DOSE
To be used to adjust for hematologic status for each cycle

WBC	PLATELETS			
	≥ 150,000	100,000–149,000	75,000–99,000	< 75,000
≥ 3,500	100%	75%	50%	0%
3,000–3,499	75%	50%	0%	0%
2,500–2,999	50%*	0%	0%	0%
< 2,500	0%	0%	0%	0%

*Delay initiation of cycle by one week if adjusted dose is below 75% of calculated dose. If adjusted dose is still below the 75% level at the third week, consult the study chairperson before treating at 50% level or allowing a 3-week delay.

Drug Combination: _____ POCC _____   Subcycle: __A__

Drug: _____ PROCARBAZINE _____

[Change Table Format?]

[Delete Table?]

WBC (x 1000)	Platelets (x 1000)			
	>= 150	100 - 150	75 - 100	< 75
>= 3.5	100% of STD	75% of STD	Delay	Delay
3.0 - 3.5	75% of STD	Delay	Delay	Delay
2.5 - 3.0	Delay	Delay	Delay	Delay
< 2.5	Delay	Delay	Delay	Delay

[Specify Abort Info]   [Specify Delay Info]

Figure 13.5. Drug dosage attenuation tables. **(Top)** The table from Northern California Oncology Group protocol 20-83-1 shows the required drug-dosage attenuations for bone-marrow toxicity. **(Bottom)** OPAL reproduces the same table on the computer screen in a manner readily understandable to physicians. The highlighted choice indicates that when a patient's white blood cell count is greater than or equal to 3500 and the platelet count is between 100,000 and 150,000, seventy-five percent of the standard dose of procarbazine should be administered.

Alterations for Lab Tests

TEST:

Hematology	Chemistries	Miscellaneous
CBC and PLTs	Alkaline Phosphatase	DLCO
CBC and PLT w/dif.	Bilirubin	ECG
Granulocytes	BUN	Pulm. Function
Hematocrit	Creatinine Clearance	
Hemoglobin	Serum Creatinine	
Platelets	SGOT	
PT	SGPT	

Selected Test: Serum Creatinine

Test Alterations for Chemotherapy: _____VAM_____   **Subcycle:** _____

Value	Action	Value	Action
_____	_____	_____	_____
_____	_____	_____	_____
_____	_____	_____	_____
_____	_____	_____	_____

Test Alterations for Drug: ___METHOTREXATE___   **(You must select a chemotherapy first)**

Value	Action	Value	Action
> 1.5	Withhold	_____	_____
_____	_____	_____	_____
_____	_____	_____	_____
_____	_____	_____	_____

Figure 13.6. Inferential knowledge in OPAL. The blanks in this form allow the expert to specify how the results of laboratory tests should cause modification of the protocol. The knowledge is automatically converted to rules for execution by ONCOCIN.

duction rule: "*If* creatinine is greater than 1.5, *then* omit the drug." The rule is applicable only within a specific context—when giving a drug (methotrexate) in a particular chemotherapy (VAM) in some protocol. As in Figure 13.4, the context is determined from the sequence of operations by which the user invoked the OPAL form and is used by OPAL to store the rule in the proper location in the ONCOCIN knowledge base.

For each class of factors that can cause protocol modifications (e.g., abnormal laboratory tests, clinical signs of toxicity), the system uses a separate form to allow the user to define the relation between specific conditions and corresponding actions. As a result, knowledge entry is organized according to the topics represented by the various forms in OPAL.

Discussion

The problems of knowledge acquisition reflect both the pitfalls of formalizing knowledge that may be poorly conceptualized and the communication difficulties that beset knowledge engineers and domain experts when neither truly understands the others' task. In the case of the original version of ONCOCIN, which was developed without OPAL, the knowledge of oncology treatment plans was already partially formalized in protocol documents. Nevertheless, the traditional communication problems of knowledge engineering remained. Building the original version of the system, which contained the knowledge of 23 similar protocols for lymphoma, required nearly 2 years and some 800 hours of an oncology fellow's time. Adding three more protocols for the adjuvant chemotherapy of breast cancer took several additional months. The length of time required to develop clinically acceptable knowledge bases could be traced to the ambiguity in the protocol documents and to the judgmental knowledge with which practicing oncologists tend to supplement the written protocol guidelines.[18]

OPAL was developed to streamline knowledge acquisition for ONCOCIN by allowing expert oncologists to enter new protocols by themselves. An important design goal in OPAL was to present a model of oncology knowledge intuitive to expert oncologists. In general, knowledge acquisition is facilitated when a knowledge engineer (or computer-based equivalent) can adopt a formal model of the application area that approximates the mental model used by the expert in everyday practice.[19]

The importance of attempting to match the conceptual model used by experts can best be related by means of an example. AI/RHEUM[20] is a rule-based consultation program for diagnosis in rheumatology, developed at the University of Missouri with the EXPERT[21] knowledge-based system building tool. The prototype version of AI/RHEUM represented knowledge directly as production rules. The early system was characterized as "completely unworkable" because "only the experts who had actually worked on the model could understand the logic."[22]

It turns out that rheumatologists often think about diagnosis in terms of the major and minor manifestations associated with particular diseases. For example, the diagnosis of rheumatic fever is customarily based on five major criteria and three minor criteria. The presence of either two of the major criteria or one major and two minor criteria indicates a high probability of rheumatic fever.[23] The first version of AI/RHEUM was "unworkable" because many physicians could not conceptualize diagnosis in rheumatology in terms of if–then rules. Knowledge acquisition was greatly facilitated when the system was rewritten so that diagnostic knowledge could be encoded as tables of major and minor criteria.[22]

In a similar manner, OPAL attempts to approximate the mental model used by expert oncologists in thinking about cancer protocols. Although no formal psychological studies were done to elicit conceptual models from physicians, the graphic displays used in OPAL for knowledge entry were designed to mimic the tables and diagrams found in oncology protocol documents. It was assumed that because the forms in OPAL were similar in organization to portions of the printed documents, OPAL's model of the domain would be perspicuous to expert oncologists. (Indeed, the anecdotal evidence suggests that oncologists can learn to work with OPAL's visual representations almost immediately.)

Cognitive psychologists maintain that the more a computer program's model of a problem approximates the mental model of the user, the easier it is for the user to tell the computer what it is he or she wants to do.[24] Therefore OPAL's model of the oncology domain is central in providing a knowledge acquisition environment that physicians can use without needing to rely on knowledge engineers for additional interpretation. At the same time, OPAL offers oncologists a visual language with a precise set of terms and relations by which protocol knowledge can be explicitly defined.

The graphic mechanisms provided in OPAL to facilitate entry of existing cancer protocols can also be used by oncologists in the design of new clinical trials. OPAL can thus be viewed not only as a knowledge-acquisition environment but also as a potential tool to assist in the development of new clinical studies.

For years, graphic interfaces that reflect strong domain models have allowed printed circuits, newspaper layouts, and various mechanical devices to be designed and fabricated automatically by domain experts working alone. In an analogous fashion, graphics-based programs such as OPAL can permit computer-aided design (CAD) of knowledge bases for expert systems without the direct need for traditional knowledge engineers. CAD systems anticipate the design problems inherent in some particular creative process, providing application-specific mechanisms to help in the refinement of plans for whatever is being designed.

The CAD systems best offset their large development costs when the design process being automated is (1) labor intensive, (2) not tolerant of errors, and (3) repetitively applied to similar problems. The development of knowledge bases for advice systems such as ONCOCIN possesses the same three features that make computer-aided design of physical objects so attractive. First, great human effort is clearly required for knowledge engineering by traditional methods. Second, whereas protocols for clinical research must be free of errors and ambiguities to be internally valid, many clinical studies appear to have significant design flaws. Encoding protocols for an expert system demands identification and resolution of unclear specifications.[18] Third, new clinical trials are constantly being developed, based on previous experimental findings. Knowledge acquisition in the ONCOCIN domain is thus an inherently repetitive process. One should be able to exploit the consistency of structure from protocol to protocol in order to facilitate knowledge entry for successive treatment plans.

The use of OPAL as an authoring environment for new knowledge bases could permit dissemination of cancer-treatment protocols in the form of *expert systems* with precise knowledge bases, rather than as text documents that may be ambiguous or misinterpreted by individual physicians. Just as OPAL can assist in the transmission of oncology protocols, analogous tools tailored for different clinical specialties also have the potential to facilitate creation and distribution of protocol knowledge bases. Recently, a program called PROTÉGÉ has been developed to generate special-purpose tools like OPAL automatically;[25] physicians in disciplines other than oncology can use these PROTÉGÉ-generated tools to enter knowledge about clinical trials in their own particular specialty. The visual metaphors first explored in OPAL can consequently facilitate the authoring of a wide spectrum of patient-care protocols. By applying principles of computer-aided design to the construction of new protocol knowledge bases, tools based on OPAL could have important benefits for clinical research.

Acknowledgments. This work has been supported by grants LM-04420, LM-07033, and RR-01631 from the National Institutes of Health. Computer facilities were provided by the SUMEX-AIM resource under NIH grant RR-00785 and through gifts from Xerox Corporation and Corning Medical. Drs. Musen and Shortliffe have also received support from the Henry J. Kaiser Family Foundation. We thank Janice Rohn, Christopher Lane, Rick Lenon, Joel Bernstein, Robert Carlson, and Charlotte Jacobs for their evaluations of the developing system.

References

1. Buchanan BG, Barstow D, Bechtal R, Bennett J, Clancey W, Kulikowski C, Mitchell T, Waterman DA: Constructing an expert system. p. 127. In Hayes-Roth F, Waterman DA, Lenat DB (eds): Building Expert Systems. Reading, MA: Addison-Wesley, 1983.
2. Tuhrim S, Reggia JA: Feasibility of physician-developed expert systems, Med Decis Making 6:23, 1986.
3. Mars NJI, Miller PL: Knowledge acquisition and verification tools for medical expert systems. Med Decis Making 7(1):6, 1987.
4. Boose JH: A knowledge acquisition program for expert systems based on personal construct psychology. Int J Man-Machine Stud 23:495, 1985.
5. Bennett JS: ROGET: a knowledge-based system for acquiring the conceptual structure of a diagnostic expert system. Automated Reasoning 1(1):49, 1985.
6. Davis R: Interactive transfer of expertise: acquisition of new inference rules. Artif Intell 12:121, 1979.
7. Politakis P, Weiss SM: Using empirical analysis to refine expert system knowledge bases. Artif Intell 22:23, 1984.

8. Shortliffe EH, Scott AC, Bischoff MB, van Melle W, Jacobs CD: ONCOCIN: an expert system for oncology protocol management. p. 876. In: Proceedings of the Seventh International Joint Conference on Artificial Intelligence, Vancouver, 1981.

9. Hickam DH, Shortliffe EH, Bischoff MB, Scott AC, Jacobs CD: A study of the treatment advice of a computer-based cancer chemothcrapy protocol advisor. Ann Intern Med 101:928, 1985.

10. Musen MA, Fagan LM, Combs DM, Shortliffe EH: Facilitating knowledge entry for an oncology therapy advisor using a model of the application area. p. 46. In: Proceedings of MEDINFO 86. Fifth World Congress on Medical Informatics, Washington, DC, 1986.

11. Musen MA, Fagan LM, Combs DM, Shortliffe EH: Use of a domain model to drive an interactive knowledge-editing tool. Int J Man-Machine Stud 26:105, 1987.

12. Musen MA, Fagan LM, Shortliffe EH: Graphical specification of procedural knowledge for an expert system. p. 15. In Hendler J (ed): Expert Systems: The User Interface, Norwood, NJ: Ablex, 1988.

13. Musen MA, Langlotz CP, Fagan LM, Shortliffe EH: Rationale for knowledge base redesign in a medical advice system. p. 197. In: Proceedings of AAMSI Congress 85. San Francisco: American Association for Medical Systems and Informatics, 1985.

14. Kahn MG, Ferguson JC, Shortliffe EH, Fagan LM: Representation and use of temporal information in ONCOCIN. p. 172. In Ackerman MJ (ed): Proceedings of the Ninth Annual Symposium on Computer Applications in Medical Care. Baltimore: IEEE Computer Society, 1985.

15. Lane CD, Walton JD, Shortliffe EH: Graphical access to medical expert systems. II. Design of an interface for physicians. Methods Inf Med 25:143, 1986.

16. Raeder G: A survey of current graphical programming techniques. Computer 18(8):11, 1985.

17. Combs DM, Musen MA, Fagan LM, Shortliffe EH: Graphical specification of procedural and inferential knowledge. p. 298. In Proceedings of AAMSI Congress 86. Anaheim, CA: American Association for Medical Systems and Informatics, 1986.

18. Musen MA, Rohn JA, Fagan LM, Shortliffe EH: Knowledge engineering for a clinical trial advice system: uncovering errors in protocol specification. p. 24. In Proceedings of AAMSI Congress 86. Anaheim, CA: American Association for Medical Systems and Informatics, 1986.

19. Gruber T, Cohen P: Design for acquisition: principles of knowledge system design to facilitate knowledge acquisition. Int J Man-Machine Stud 26:143, 1987.

20. Lindberg DAB, Sharp GC, Kingsland LC, Weiss SM, Hayes SP, Ueno H, Hazelwood SE: Computer based rheumatology consultant. p. 1311. In: Proceedings MEDINFO 80. Third World Conference of Medical Informatics. Amsterdam: North Holland, 1980.

21. Weiss SM, Kulikowski CA: EXPERT: a system for developing consultation models. p. 942. In: Proceedings of the Sixth International Joint Conference on Artificial Intelligence, Tokyo, 1979.

22. Lindberg DAB, Kingsland LC, Roeseler DR, Sharp GC: A new knowledge representation for diagnosis in rheumatology. p. 299. In: Proceedings: AMIA

Congress 82. San Francisco: American Association for Medical Systems and Informatics, 1982.
23. Stollerman GH, Markowitz M, Taranta A, Wanamaker LW, Whittemore R: Jones criteria (revised) for guidance in the diagnosis of rheumatic fever. Circulation 32:664, 1965.
24. Norman DA: Cognitive engineering. p. 31. In Norman DA, Draper SW (eds): User Centered System Design. Hillsdale, NJ: Erlbaum, 1986.
25. Musen MA: Generation of Model-Based Knowledge-Acquisition Tools for Clinical-Trial Advice Systems. Ph.D. Thesis, Stanford University, Report STAN-CS-88-1194, 1988.

14
HYDRA: A Knowledge Acquisition Tool for Expert Systems That Critique Medical Work-up

Perry L. Miller, Steven J. Blumenfrucht,
John R. Rose, Michael Rothschild,
Henry A. Swett, Gregory Weltin, and
Nicolaas J.I. Mars

When constructing an expert consultation system to give computer-based advice to the practicing physician, a major problem arises in ensuring that the system's knowledge of its domain is well organized, accurate, complete, and consistent. Even in a constrained domain, the knowledge base typically becomes so complex that the system builders cannot be expected to recall in detail its exact contents or to anticipate all the ways the knowledge might interact. As a result, there is an urgent need to develop tools that allow the computer itself to assist in creating and verifying such a knowledge base.

HYDRA is a knowledge acquisition tool under development to assist in the creation of expert systems that critique medical work-up. Medical work-up involves performing a sequence of specific tests to explore a particular medical problem. At each point in the work-up sequence, the best test typically depends on the patient and the results of tests already performed. Work-up is a focused process that occurs after initial differential diagnosis has proposed a set of possible diagnoses a patient may have.

To use HYDRA, as illustrated in Figure 14.1, a domain expert first outlines the recommended work-up approach, expressed using the augmented transition network (ATN) formalism. As described later in the chapter, this ATN model indicates the recommended sequences of tests, together with the conditions under which each test is preferred. From the ATN model, HYDRA produces a list of the various conditions for which critiquing comments may be required to allow an expert system to critique work-up in that domain. These comments are used by that system, as illustrated later, to react to all correct and erroneous approaches that might be proposed.

The list of conditions HYDRA produces is designed to simplify the knowledge acquisition process. Using HYDRA, the domain expert need not worry about the global structure of the critiquing system being built.

Adapted from Miller PL, Blumenfrucht SJ, Rose JR et al: HYDRA: A knowledge acquisition tool for expert systems which critique medical workup. *Medical Decision Making* 7:12–21, 1987. Reprinted with permission.

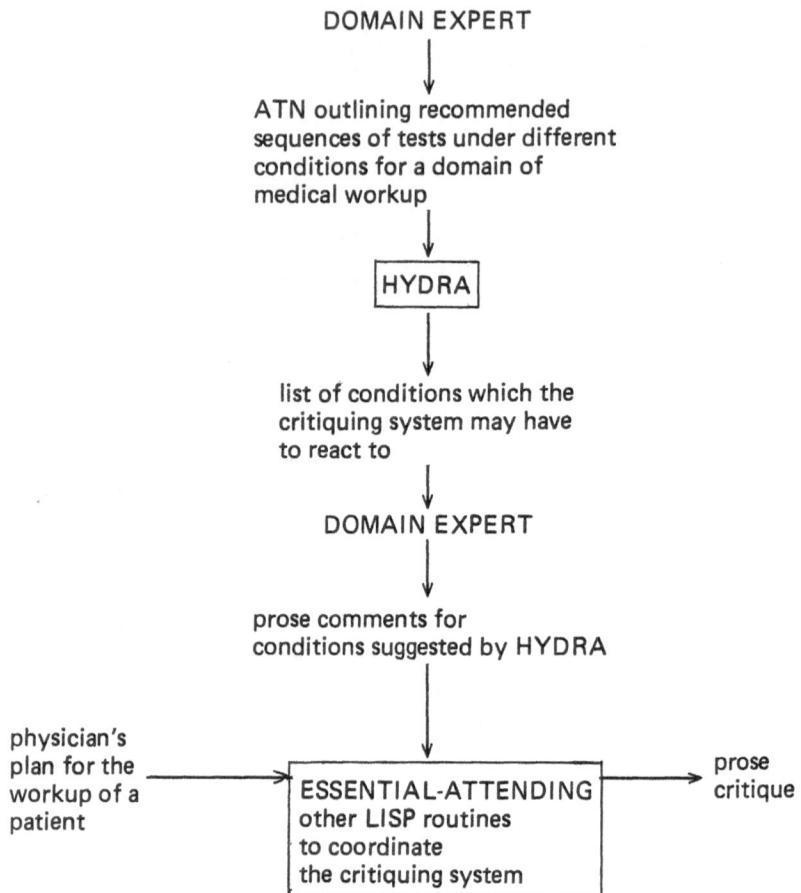

Figure 14.1 Outline of how HYDRA helps a domain expert build an expert critiquing system for a chosen domain of medical work-up.

An organized, hierarchical design is automatically provided. The domain expert can therefore be concerned primarily with constructing and polishing a set of well defined prose comments. In addition, it must be ascertained that these comments are phrased so that the overall thread of thought flows smoothly in the ultimate critique.

Critiquing

Several previous systems have explored the critiquing approach to bringing computer-based advice to the practicing physician. They include systems in domains of medical management,[1-4] work-up,[5] and differential diagnosis.[6] Whereas the traditional expert system attempts to tell a physician how to approach the patient's care, a critiquing system first asks the physician what approach is being contemplated and then critiques that plan. It is anticipated that the critiquing approach is particularly well suited for domains where decisions involve a considerable amount of subjective judgment.

From the experience gained implementing these systems, a system-building system, ESSENTIAL-ATTENDING, has been developed to facilitate the implementation of critiquing systems.[7] Prototype systems have already been implemented using ESSENTIAL-ATTENDING in areas of medical management, work-up, and differential diagnosis.

A central component of ESSENTIAL-ATTENDING is the "expressive frame" containing sets of critiquing comments that react to the various parts of the physician's plan. Each comment includes the *condition* under which that comment is to be included in the system's critique. An example condition would be "if an ultrasound test is ordered (for initial work-up of obstructive jaundice) and the patient is massively obese and not allergic to contrast medium." The critiquing comment for this condition would discuss in detail why ultrasound is not appropriate in this situation and why a computed tomography (CT) scan is preferred.

HYDRA's task is to take the ATN that outlines recommended work-up in a particular domain and from that ATN produce a list of all conditions that might require such critiquing comments. In this way, HYDRA breaks the domain expert's work into a set of small, fairly independent, easily understood tasks.

DxCON: An Example Critiquing System for Obstructive Jaundice

The various components of HYDRA's design are discussed later in the chapter. To help make that description more easily understood, this section first shows an example system critiquing medical work-up. Specifically, this section demonstrates DxCON, a system under development to critique the radiologic work-up of obstructive jaundice. (The obstructive jaundice domain is used throughout the chapter to illustrate HYDRA's various features.)

As shown in Figure 14.2, five diagnostic tests may be used in the work-up of suspected obstructive jaundice.

1. After initial data are gathered, an ultrasound (US) examination is usually the first imaging test performed. In certain circumstances, however, a CT scan is indicated instead.
2. If either of these initial tests produces unsatisfactory results, the other may be done.
3. If the biliary ducts are not seen to be dilated, a radionuclide study (HIDA) may still be able to document biliary obstruction.
4. Depending on the results of this initial work-up, the next step may involve medical treatment, surgical treatment, or further work-up using

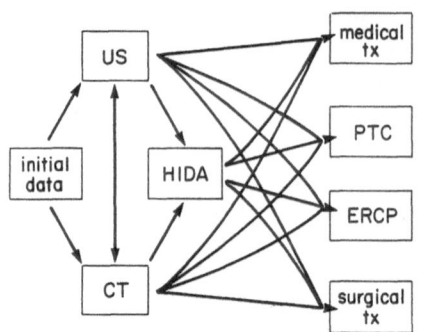

Figure 14.2. Outline of the work-up of obstructive jaundice in an abbreviated flow chart form.

either percutaneous transhepatic cholangiography (PTC) or endoscopic retrograde cholangiopancreatography (ERCP).

Thus the work-up of obstructive jaundice involves sequencing a subset of five tests (US, CT, HIDA, PTC, and ERCP), with various considerations as to which test is most appropriate at each decision point. There is also latitude for practice variation in certain patients, which makes the critiquing approach particularly appropriate.

The example shown below illustrates DxCON in operation. Here, for the initial work-up of a patient with suspected obstructive jaundice, a physician has suggested a CT scan. The patient is massively obese and allergic to intravenous contrast material. The patient and the proposed plan are described to the system, which responds with the following critique.

> The radiologic investigation of suspected obstructive jaundice generally proceeds from noninvasive, inexpensive tests to invasive, expensive ones. History, physical examination, and laboratory tests are assumed to be completed and to suggest obstructive jaundice. Other conditions such as cholecystitis and medical jaundice are therefore not considered further by this program.
>
> The noninvasive tests available for the evaluation of jaundice include ultrasound (US), computed tomography (CT), and radionuclide scintigraphy (HIDA). Generally, a structural study (US or CT) is performed prior to any other test. These tests are noninvasive and usually yield the most information in the least time. They systematically survey a large area of the body and are therefore useful as initial screening examinations.
>
> Ultrasound is generally preferred to CT for the initial evaluation of suspected obstructive jaundice because of its low cost, portability, and excellent sensitivity for biliary dilatation, gallstones, hepatic masses, and pancreatic pathology. In a massively obese patient, however, the US examination is frequently limited and CT is usually preferred. If, on the other hand, the patient is also allergic to intravenous contrast material, US may be the better initial choice. (If the US study does turn out to be unsatisfactory, it may be followed by a noncontrast CT scan or even by a contrast CT scan if the patient is appropriately premedicated.)

The critique starts off with a variety of *introductory material* discussing: (1) the work-up of obstructive jaundice in general (paragraph 1); (2) non-invasive tests (paragraph 2, sentence 1); (3) initial tests (paragraph 2, sentences 2 to 4); and (4) the use of a CT scan as an initial test (paragraph 3, sentences 1 and 2). The critique then comments on the *indications* and *contraindications* of the CT scan for the patient described. Because the work-up process is just starting, no further discussion is included. Had the patient's work-up been further along, the critique might have included a discussion of the results of any tests performed and the implications of those results for further work-up.

The remainder of this chapter describes how HYDRA is designed to assist in constructing a system to produce such a critique. The critiquing approach itself and its motivation are described in more detail elsewhere.[1-7]

Using the ATN to Build a Parallel Model of the Domain

To use HYDRA, the system builder must first construct a model of the domain using the ATN formalism. Using a general model of the work-up process is possible because most nontrivial domains of work-up do indeed have a similar structure: a sequence of tests where the best next test depends on the patient and on previous tests. Figure 14.3 shows an example ATN that models the recommended work-up of obstructive jaundice.

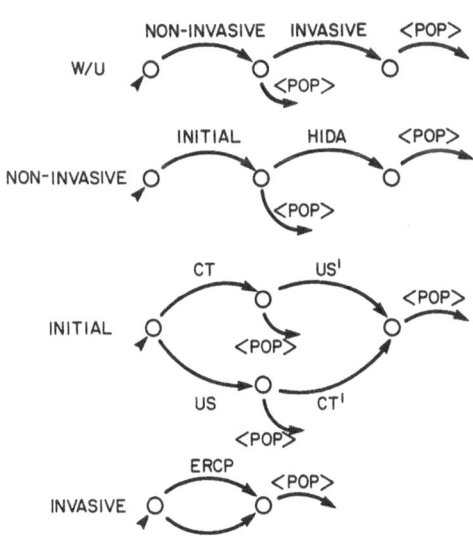

Figure 14.3. Outline of the work-up of obstructive jaundice in ATN form.

Structure of the ATN

The ATN model is hierarchical, with different networks representing levels of decision and subdecision. Thus at the "topmost" level (in the W/U network), NONINVASIVE tests are followed by INVASIVE tests. Lower-level ATN networks then indicate how NONINVASIVE and INVASIVE work-up should be performed. NONINVASIVE work-up consists of INITIAL work-up, followed possibly by a HIDA scan. INITIAL work-up consists of either a CT or US test, followed possibly by the other.

Each ATN network consists of *states* (circles) connected by *arcs*. Each arc is labeled either with the name of a specific *test* (US, CT) or a *class* of tests (NONINVASIVE, INITIAL). As shown in Figure 14.4, many arcs have associated conditions indicating when those arcs should be used. Thus in the INITIAL network the CT arc should be used if the patient is massively obese and not allergic to contrast material. Otherwise, a US test should be performed.

Starting from the *initial state* of a network, preferred work-up is defined by tracing a *path* from state to state along the arcs. The path in a network ends whenever a *pop* arc is used. Whenever an arc is taken that is labeled with the name of a test class (e.g., INITIAL), processing halts temporarily while a path is traced through the lower network, after which processing of the higher network resumes. The conditions associated with the arcs indicate when the associated test should be used in the recommended

```
CT arc condition

    (AND (PATIENT OBESE)(NOT (PATIENT ALLERGY CONTRAST)))

CT' arc condition

    (OR (US UNSATISFACTORY)(US STONE QUESTION)
        (US MASS QUESTION)(US DUCT-DILATATION QUESTION))

US' arc condition

    (OR (CT UNSATISFACTORY)(CT STONE QUESTION)
        (CT MASS QUESTION)(CT DUCT-DILATATION QUESTION))

HIDA arc condition

    (OR  (AND (NOT (US DONE))(CT DUCT-DILATATION NO))
         (AND (NOT (CT DONE))(US DUCT-DILATATION NO))
         (AND (US DUCT-DILATATION NO)(CT DUCT-DILATATION YES))
         (AND (CT DUCT-DILATATION NO)(US DUCT-DILATATION YES))
         (AND (US DUCT-DILATATION NO)(CT DUCT-DILATATION QUESTION))
         (AND (US DUCT-DILATATION NO)(CT DUCT-DILATATION NO))
         (AND (US DUCT-DILATATION QUESTION)(CT DUCT-DILATATION NO))
         (AND (US DUCT-DILATATION QUESTION)(CT DUCT-DILATATION QUESTION)))

INVASIVE arc condition

    (AND (HIDA INDICATED)(HIDA OBSTRUCTION NO))
```

Figure 14.4. List of the various conditions associated with arcs of the ATN shown in Figure 14.3. (The INVASIVE arc condition has been simplified.)

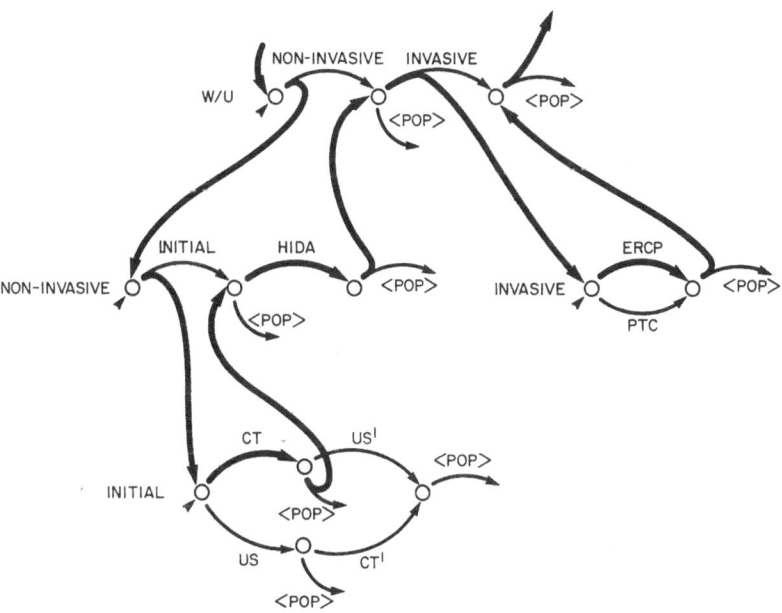

Figure 14.5. Path through the entire ATN that corresponds to a complete work-up sequence.

work-up sequence. As illustrated in Figure 14.5, a path through the entire network corresponds to a complete recommended work-up sequence.

It is instructive to compare the ATN model (Fig. 14.3) with the flow chart model shown in Figure 14.2. The main difference is that the ATN model is hierarchical, which has several advantages.

1. The ATN model forces the domain expert to conceptualize the domain in hierarchical terms. As discussed later, the hierarchical model helps give the critiquing system a useful, organized structure.
2. Another advantage of the hierarchical model is that paths which diverge in a lower network later rejoin when the path returns to a higher network. For example, no matter which INITIAL test sequence is performed, the various paths always rejoin in the NONINVASIVE network before proceeding to HIDA. Similarly, all NONINVASIVE paths rejoin before proceeding to INVASIVE tests. As discussed later, this structure makes it easy for the results of a related set of tests to be discussed together if the system designer chooses. This hierarchical model contrasts with the flow chart model, where one can go directly from virtually any of the early tests to any later test. As a result, the flow chart is not as clean a framework around which to structure the knowledge acquisition process.

Structuring Knowledge Acquisition Using HYDRA

The ATN model of a work-up domain serves two important purposes.

1. It is used to drive the knowledge acquisition process. This use of the ATN is described in this section.
2. It is used to provide an organized hierarchical structure for the prose critique itself. This use of the ATN is described later in the chapter.

Once the ATN model is defined, the knowledge acquisition process involves three more steps: (1) completing the ATN; (2) listing a set of conditions for critiquing comments; and (3) iterative refinement of the ATN model.

Completing the ATN

Once an ATN model has been constructed for a chosen work-up domain, the next step involves adding "bypass" arcs to the ATN. These arcs correspond to paths where tests should have been performed but were not, as shown in Figure 14.6. The arcs of the original ATN represent either specific tests (US, CT) or classes of tests (NONINVASIVE, INITIAL). Comparing Figure 14.6 with Figure 14.3, one sees several added "bypass" arcs: (NO NONINVASIVE), (NO INITIAL), (NO HIDA), etc. These

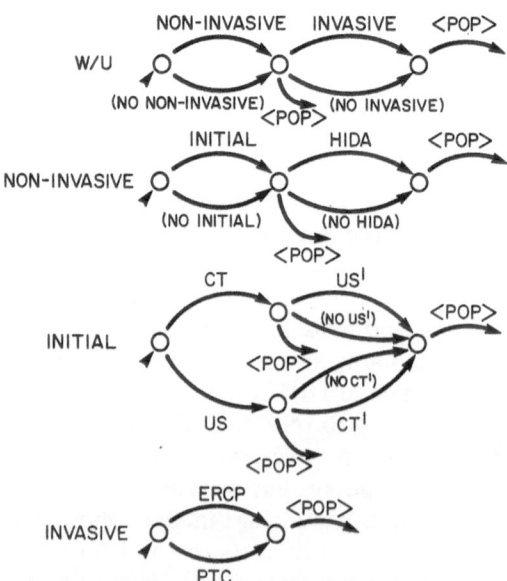

Figure 14.6. Obstructive jaundice ATN with "bypass" arcs added corresponding to tests that should have been performed but were not.

arcs are currently added by hand, although a later version of HYDRA might add them automatically.

The new network contains a path for any possible set of tests. The new network does not, however, allow all possible nonrecommended sequences of tests, nor does it allow a test to be repeated. These two issues are discussed later in the chapter.

Listing Conditions for Critiquing Comments

The next step involves producing a set of suggested conditions for which critiquing comments should be written by the domain expert. Such a list is compiled for each of the following:

1. Each *test* listed in the ATN
2. Each *test class* listed in the ATN
3. Each *bypass* arc added to the ATN, as described earlier in the chapter.

The following example illustrates how it is done. The CT arc in the INITIAL network has the following associated condition:

```
(AND (PATIENT OBESE)
     (NOT (PATIENT ALLERGY CONTRAST)))
```

This condition (expressed as a data structure in the LISP programming language) states that the CT arc should be taken only if the patient is massively obese and not allergic to intravenous contrast material. For this arc, HYDRA suggests the following conditions, which may require comment when the actual work-up sequence starts with a CT scan.

```
Comment: Introduction to CT
Comment: (AND (PATIENT OBESE)
              (NOT (PATIENT ALLERGY CONTRAST)))
Comment: (AND (PATIENT OBESE)
              (PATIENT ALLERGY CONTRAST))
Comment: (AND (NOT (PATIENT OBESE))
              (NOT (PATIENT ALLERGY CONTRAST)))
Comment: (AND (NOT (PATIENT OBESE))
              (PATIENT ALLERGY CONTRAST))
Comment: Any other conditions affecting CT that merit discussion
Comment: Any results of CT that merit discussion
```

Thus HYDRA suggests (1) an introductory comment discussing the use of CT as an initial test, (2) four comments derived from the arc's condition discussing the different possible appropriate and inappropriate uses of the test, (3) any further conditions for which the domain expert wants to include comments regarding the test, and (4) any results of the test the domain expert wants discussed.

Below are the comments the domain expert has entered into DxCON for this arc:

1. *Introductory comment:* "Ultrasound is generally preferred to CT for the initial evaluation of suspected obstructive jaundice because of its low cost, portability, and excellent sensitivity for biliary dilatation, gallstones, hepatic masses, and pancreatic pathology."

2. *Comment (obese, no allergy):* "In a massively obese patient, however, the US examination is frequently limited and CT is usually preferred. (Note, however, that if the patient's weight exceeds the limit for the CT table, typically 275 to 300 pounds, a CT cannot be performed.)"

3. *Comment (obese, allergy):* "In a massively obese patient, however, the US examination is frequently limited and CT is usually preferred. If, on the other hand, the patient is also allergic to intravenous contrast material, US may be the better initial choice. (If the US study does turn out to be unsatisfactory, it may be followed by a noncontrast CT scan or even by a contrast CT scan if the patient is appropriately premedicated.)"

4. *Comment (not obese):* "In a massively obese patient, the US examination is frequently limited, and CT is therefore preferred. In a patient who is not massively obese, however, we see no reason to prefer CT as an initial study."

5. *Comment (obese and NPO):* "If a patient is NPO and cannot take oral contrast material, CT is less useful because it may be difficult to differentiate bowel from abnormal masses. Useful diagnostic information is nevertheless obtained, especially in areas not usually confused with bowel, e.g., hepatic parenchyma. Therefore if CT is otherwise indicated, we normally recommend that it be done even if the patient is NPO."

Note that two conditions suggested by HYDRA involving [NOT (PATIENT OBESE)] have been collapsed into a *single* comment (comment 4). (See the discussion of constraints, below.) Also, one additional comment has been included for use if the patient is NPO. Note also that no comments are included to discuss CT results. As described below, the domain expert can choose where in the hierarchy of tests and test classes the results of a given test are discussed. The results of CT can be discussed after CT itself is discussed, after all initial tests are discussed, or after all noninvasive tests have been discussed. In DxCON, the results of all noninvasive tests are discussed as a unit, in the comments associated with the NONINVASIVE arc.

Iterative Refinement of the ATN Model

Once the ATN model has been defined and a set of conditions has been suggested by HYDRA for critiquing comments, there may well be a period of iterative refinement as the ATN or its conditions are modified. Also, it may be deemed necessary to incorporate *constraints* into the ATN model, as discussed later.

We anticipate that the initial definition of the ATN and its refinement will usually *not* be performed solely by the domain expert. Rather, it will be done in close collaboration with a knowledge engineer familiar with the HYDRA system. (A *knowledge engineer* is a computer specialist familiar with the construction and refinement of expert knowledge bases.) If the domain expert is unfamiliar with computer technology, the knowledge engineer may well carry out all the actual interaction with HYDRA.

Once the refinement of the ATN is complete and a satisfactory set of conditions for critiquing comments are produced, the domain expert can then work on his own to construct and polish the set of comments. These initial comments may, of course, require later revision as the system is refined using test cases.

Hierarchical Structure of the Critique

Figure 14.7 outlines the order in which critiquing comments are listed for the domain expert. This order reflects the hierarchical structure of the ATN model. Indeed, the list is compiled by tracing paths through the ATN. It is also the same order in which the comments will appear in the prose critique. The prose critique, of course, contains only those comments that apply to the patient described.

As demonstrated in Figure 14.7, the set of comments for *test classes* are split in three parts.

1. For each test class, HYDRA first requests an introductory comment, comments regarding indications, and additional comments.
2. HYDRA then requests comments for all subclasses and subtests in the test class.
3. Finally, HYDRA requests comments discussing the results of the test class.

The domain expert may therefore indicate that the results of a test be discussed at any chosen level of the hierarchy. Indeed, in our experience it appears useful to discuss all the results of closely related tests as a unit. The hierarchical structure makes it clear to the domain expert how it can be done.

Constraints to Restrict the Conditions
Suggested for Comments

As mentioned previously, HYDRA allows the system builder to specify *constraints* that restrict the number of conditions listed by HYDRA for critiquing comments. Each such constraint is stored with the ATN arc to which the constraint applies.

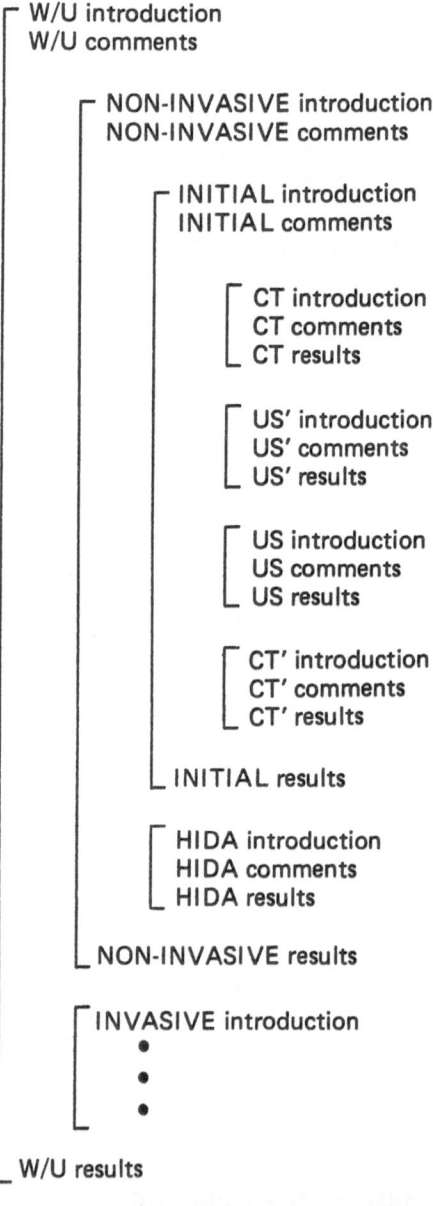

Figure 14.7. Outline of the order in which conditions for critiquing comments are listed. This is the same order in which the comments will appear in the prose critique. The comments are indented to reflect the underlying hierarchical structure which mirrors that of the ATN. (For clarity, comments associated with bypass arcs are not included. They directly follow the comments associated with the test or test class that is bypassed.)

Constraints: A Simple Example

A simple constraint is as follows:

Name: NOT-OBESE
Justification: If the patient is not massively obese, allergy to contrast material is irrelevant.
Description: IF (NOT (PATIENT OBESE))
                IGNORE (PATIENT ALLERGY CONTRAST)

A constraint has three components.

1. *Constraint name:* The choice of a name is arbitrary. Constraint names allow the system builder to relax (deactivate) constraints selectively if desired.
2. *Prose justification:* Each constraint may also have an associated prose justification. Whenever the constraint is used by HYDRA to restrict a set of suggested conditions, this justification is available to explain why the constraint was used.
3. *Functional description of the constraint:* Each constraint also has a functional description. For example, the description above indicates that "when a suggested condition includes (NOT (PATIENT OBESE)) *and* (PATIENT ALLERGY CONTRAST), HYDRA can disregard whether the condition (PATIENT ALLERGY CONTRAST) holds.

Using the NOT-OBESE constraint shown above when processing the CT arc condition:

    (AND (PATIENT OBESE)
         (NOT (PATIENT ALLERGY CONTRAST)))

results in the following *three* conditions suggested by HYDRA for possible critiquing comments.

    1. (AND (PATIENT OBESE)
            (NOT (PATIENT ALLERGY CONTRAST)))
    2. (AND (PATIENT OBESE)
            (PATIENT ALLERGY CONTRAST))
    3. (NOT (PATIENT OBESE)

If the system builder then asks that the constraint "NOT-OBESE" be relaxed (deactivated), then *four* conditions are suggested.

    1. (AND (PATIENT OBESE)
            (NOT (PATIENT ALLERGY CONTRAST))
    2. (AND (PATIENT OBESE)
            (PATIENT ALLERGY CONTRAST))
    3. (AND (NOT (PATIENT OBESE)
            (NOT (PATIENT ALLERGY CONTRAST)))
    4. (AND (NOT (PATIENT OBESE))
            (PATIENT ALLERGY CONTRAST))

The constraint therefore implies that conditions 3 and 4 can be collapsed into a single condition and handled by a single critiquing comment. This constraint represents a judgment made by the domain expert regarding the domain.

Constraints: A More Complex Example

A more complex example may make the need for constraints more apparent. As shown in Figure 14.4, a HIDA scan is indicated for the work-up of obstructive jaundice when initial tests are negative or questionable. The actual combination of conditions under which HIDA may be indicated is reasonably complex.

```
(OR (AND (NOT (CT DONE))
         (CT DUCT-DILATATION NO))
    (AND (NOT (CT DONE))
         (US DUCT-DILATATION NO))
    (AND (US DUCT-DILATATION NO)
         (CT DUCT-DILATATION YES))
    (AND (CT DUCT-DILATATION NO)
         (US DUCT-DILATATION YES))
    (AND (US DUCT-DILATATION NO)
         (CT DUCT-DILATATION QUESTION))
    (AND (US DUCT-DILATATION NO)
         (CT DUCT-DILATATION NO))
    (AND (US DUCT-DILATATION QUESTION)
         (CT DUCT-DILATAION NO))
    (AND (US DUCT-DILATATION QUESTION)
         (CT DUCT-DILATATION QUESTION))
```

When this set of conditions is processed to obtain a comprehensive set of suggested conditions for critiquing comments, the list of such conditions becomes quite formidable.

```
(AND (CT DUCT-DILATATION YES)
     (NOT (US DONE)))
(AND (CT DUCT-DILATATION NO)
     (NOT (US DONE)))
(AND (CT DUCT-DILATATION UNKNOWN)
     (NOT (US DONE)))
(AND (CT DUCT-DILATATION QUESTION)
     (NOT (US DONE)))
(AND (CT DUCT-DILATATION YES)
     (US DONE))
(AND (CT DUCT-DILATATION NO)
     (US DONE))
```

```
(AND (CT DUCT-DILATATION UNKNOWN)
     (US DONE))
(AND (CT DUCT-DILATATION QUESTION)
     (US DONE))
(AND (NOT (CT DONE))
     (US DUCT-DILATATION YES))
(AND (NOT (CT DONE))
     (US DUCT-DILATATION NO))
(AND (NOT (CT DONE))
     (US DUCT-DILATATION UNKNOWN))
(AND (NOT (CT DONE))
     (US DUCT-DILATAION QUESTION))
(AND (CT DONE)
     (US DUCT-DILATATION YES))
(AND (CT DONE)
     (US DUCT-DILATATION NO))
(AND (CT DONE)
     (US DUCT-DILATATION UNKNOWN))
(AND (CT DONE)
     (US DUCT-DILATATION QUESTION))
(AND (CT DUCT-DILATATION YES)
     (US DUCT-DILATATION YES))
(AND (CT DUCT-DILATATION NO)
     (US DUCT-DILATATION YES))
(AND (CT DUCT-DILATATION UNKNOWN)
     (US DUCT-DILATATION YES))
(AND (CT DUCT-DILATATION QUESTION)
     (US DUCT-DILATATION YES))
(AND (CT DUCT-DILATATION YES)
     (US DUCT-DILATATION NO))
(AND (CT DUCT-DILATATION NO)
     (US DUCT-DILATATION NO))
(AND (CT DUCT-DILATATION UNKNOWN)
     (US DUCT-DILATATION NO))
(AND (CT DUCT-DILATATION QUESTION)
     (US DUCT-DILATATION NO))
(AND (CT DUCT-DILATATION YES)
     (US DUCT-DILATATION UNKNOWN))
(AND (CT DUCT-DILATATION NO)
     (US DUCT-DILATATION UNKNOWN))
(AND (CT DUCT-DILATATION UNKNOWN)
     (US DUCT-DILATATION UNKNOWN))
(AND (CT DUCT-DILATATION QUESTION)
     (US DUCT-DILATATION UNKNOWN))
(AND (CT DUCT-DILATATION YES)
     (US DUCT-DILATATION QUESTION))
```

```
(AND (CT DUCT-DILATATION NO)
     (US DUCT-DILATATION QUESTION))
(AND (CT DUCT-DILATATION UNKNOWN)
     (US DUCT-DILATATION QUESTION))
(AND (CT DUCT-DILATATION QUESTION)
     (US DUCT-DILATATION QUESTION))
```

It would not be very helpful for a domain expert to be presented with this list of conditions for critiquing comments. Indeed, "expressive economies" inherent in the domain presumably make separate comments for each of these conditions unnecessary. The constraint shown below captures these expressive economies. Using the constraint, the 32 conditions shown above can be reduced to *two* conditions requiring critiquing comments.

Name: HIDA-INDICATED
Justification: It is possible deal with the various conditions for which HIDA is indicated in the prose comments themselves.
Description: SUBSTITUTE (HIDA INDICATED) FOR

```
(OR (AND (NOT (US DONE))
         (CT DUCT-DILATATION NO))
    (AND (NOT (CT DONE))
         (US DUCT-DILATATION NO))
    (AND (US DUCT-DILATATION NO)
         (CT DUCT-DILATATION YES))
    (AND (CT DUCT-DILATATION NO)
         (US DUCT-DILATATION YES))
    (AND (US DUCT-DILATATION NO)
         (CT DUCT-DILATATION QUESTION))
    (AND (US DUCT-DILATATION NO)
         (CT DUCT-DILATATION NO))
    (AND (US DUCT-DILATATION QUESTION)
         (CT DUCT-DILATAION NO))
    (AND (US DUCT-DILATATION QUESTION)
         (CT DUCT-DILATATION QUESTION))
```

This constraint results in the single condition (HIDA INDICATED) being substituted for the more complex condition when processing the HIDA arc to produce a list of suggested conditions. (The substitution is performed dynamically. No permanent change is made to the arc itself.) As a result, only two conditions are suggested to the domain expert for critiquing comments.

1. (HIDA INDICATED)
2. (NOT (HIDA INDICATED))

As indicated in the constraint's prose justification, this simplification is possible because the various conditions can be handled adequately in two prose comments. Specifically, for the HIDA arc the DxCON system includes the following comments.

1. *Introductory comment:* A HIDA scan can detect the presence of biliary obstruction in the absence of biliary dilatation, which can occur in up to 10 percent of cases.

2. *If HIDA is indicated:* It is therefore a reasonable choice for this patient.

3. *If HIDA is not indicated:* In the presence of biliary tract dilatation documented by US or CT, therefore, little useful information is likely to be gained by this examination.

These comments allow DxCON to react appropriately to all conditions. In this way, the constraint might be seen to take advantage of "expressive economies" inherent in the domain.

Other Types of Constraint

HYDRA currently allows four types of constraint.

1. *Negation-only constraints:* Certain conditions have more than one alternative, e.g., a mass on US may be (1) present, (2) absent, (3) questionable, or (4) unknown. When such a condition is processed, four conditions are obtained requiring critiquing comments. When a negation-only constraint is applied, the condition generates only two conditions: itself and not itself.
2. *Conditionally-ignore constraints:* See previous example.
3. *Substitution constraints:* See previous example.
4. *Treat-class-as-unit constraints:* In some domains a certain class of tests may best be treated as a single unit and not broken down for discussion as individual tests. In DxCON, for example, PTC and ERCP are close in their clinical indications and use. Indeed, in many institutions the choice is based on local preference and expertise. As a result, DxCON discusses INVASIVE tests as a single unit and does not include separate sets of critiquing comments for PTC and ERCP individually.

As we explore the use of HYDRA in other domains, further types of constraint may well be encountered.

How Constraints Are Defined

The integration of constraints into the ATN is part of the iterative refinement process outlined earlier in the chapter. Most computer-naive domain experts would find it difficult to recognize the applicability of a constraint by themselves. We therefore anticipate that the definition of constraints is usually performed with the assistance of a knowledge engineer familiar with the HYDRA system.

Additional Design Feature: Graceful Degradation

The preceding sections have described HYDRA's principal design features. This section addresses one further issue. HYDRA is designed to structure a critique in which tests are discussed *in the order in which they should have been performed*. As a result, if the tests have been performed in a much different order, the critique may not fully capture the implications of the abnormal order, particularly with respect to the appropriateness of the later tests performed.

Two approaches could have been taken to deal with this problem. HYDRA could have been designed to construct a critiquing system to react fully to the implications of *all* (even nonsensical) permutations in sequence. This approach was not taken for several reasons. First, HYDRA would have had to ask the domain expert to prepare comments for many obscure and unlikely conditions. The approach would also have violated our main design goal: to structure the knowledge found in the clinical literature around a particular plan for a patient's care. The clinical literature usually discusses how medicine should be practiced. Although it may highlight certain important errors, it does not dwell on all the implications of every conceivable obscure, nonsensical error.

For these reasons we adopted a different approach. HYDRA is designed to help build a system that reacts appropriately to fairly normal errors and that "degrades gracefully" when presented with more unusual errors. For example, if the work-up sequence described differs radically from that recommended, DxCON includes the following disclaimer in its critique.

> DxCON sequences the comments in its critique in the same order that we normally recommend obstructive jaundice be worked up. All the implications of a significant departure from this standard order may not be fully addressed in our comments. Please bear this in mind when reading the critique.

A similar approach is taken if tests are repeated. DxCON critiques the use of the test in its recommended sequence and then adds a comment discussing the repetition of tests in general terms. (A domain expert is always free, of course, to add critiquing comments that deal with these issues in more detail.)

HYDRA: Current Status

It is important to emphasize that HYDRA is an experimental knowledge acquisition tool still undergoing refinement. It was developed primarily in conjunction with the DxCON system whose domain is obstructive jaundice. Simultaneously we have also explored several other work-up domains in sufficient depth to believe that HYDRA's general design will adapt well to a range of such domains. The system has yet to be exposed, however, to domain experts outside our group of collaborators. It is also important to emphasize that the DxCON system is a developmental system, currently undergoing evaluation and refinement as it is tested with clinical cases.

We anticipate that as we explore different domains further design issues will be encountered. One such issue is *conflicting expertise*. In many areas of medicine, there is overt disagreement between experts as to the best approach. In such domains it will be important to let the domain expert incorporate such conflicting viewpoints, if so desired, into the critiquing system and into the prose critique produced.

The incorporation of conflicting expertise into a system that critiques medical work-up has been previously explored.[5] In DxCON our domain expert did not deem it necessary to include conflicting expertise. In other domains, however, HYDRA will need to be augmented to allow conflicting expert opinions.

How HYDRA Compares to Other Approaches to Knowledge Acquisition

Several research projects have developed sophisticated computer-based tools to assist in knowledge acquisition (KA) and knowledge verification (KV) for medical expert systems. To help put HYDRA's approach into perspective, this section discusses certain of its features compared to other approaches that have been explored.

1. *Interface between HYDRA and the domain expert.* Some approaches, e.g., that of TEIRESIAS,[8] allow the domain expert to interact directly with the system in the process of KA. Although such direct interaction is certainly possible with HYDRA for a computer-sophisticated domain expert, it is anticipated that a knowledge engineer familiar with HYDRA will help the domain expert when constructing the ATN, entering it into the system, and defining any constraints, as well as with the process of iterative refinement. Once a satisfactory set of suggestions for critiquing comments is obtained, however, the domain expert can work independently to create and polish those comments.

2. *Knowledge acquisition as a vehicle to structure system design.* Some approaches to KA, such as that of TEIRESIAS, start with an existing knowledge base and attempt to help the domain expert add more knowledge. In contrast, HYDRA is designed for the initial phases of system creation. A by-product of this approach is that HYDRA is able to enforce an overall structure on the emerging knowledge base. In this respect, HYDRA is similar to OPAL,[9] which structures the initial acquisition of knowledge for oncology protocols. Using a KA tool to help build a knowl-

edge base from scratch may prove to be a valuable vehicle for enforcing the construction of well organized knowledge bases for expert systems.

3. *Using constraints to refine a general model of work-up to the unique requirements of a domain.* An interesting question in the design of KA and KV tools is how to adapt a general model of a class of domains to the unique characteristics of a particular domain. HYDRA uses the ATN to model work-up in general and allows the use of constraints to adapt this general model to a particular work-up problem. SEEK[10] adapts a general model of differential diagnosis to a particular domain using a set of test cases gathered from that domain. TEIRESIAS attempts to adapt to a domain by inferring generalizations from patterns seen in an existing knowledge base. It thereby creates expectations regarding the characteristics of knowledge in that domain.

4. *Source of the knowledge that drives KA and KV.* A common feature shared by several of the KA and KV projects is the use of what might be called a "parallel model" of the domain, in addition to the system's knowledge base.[11] For KA, this parallel model guides the incorporation of new knowledge into the knowledge base. For KV, the parallel model is used to help check the knowledge base for accuracy and completeness.

Several types of a parallel model have been used to drive the KA/KV process. (1) In TEIRESIAS *the system itself* infers a set of hypothesized generalizations from the knowledge base, which in turn guide KA and KV. (2) In SEEK, *a set of test cases* with known diagnoses are used to drive KV. (3) In OPAL, *the system builder* explicitly outlines a hierarchical model of an oncology protocol that then guides the KA process. HYDRA's approach is similar to that of OPAL, as the domain expert explicitly outlines a model of the domain.

Summary

HYDRA is a knowledge acquisition tool designed to model the process of medical work-up. The model allows a domain expert to outline the recommended work-up of a medical problem and to receive a list of the various conditions for which comments may be required to build an expert system to critique work-up in that domain.

The problem of ensuring that a knowledge base is well organized and complete is a major problem impeding the widespread application of expert system technology. There is a real need for computer-based tools that can help the domain expert with this problem. HYDRA demonstrates one way such a tool might be designed. Indeed HYDRA defines a structure and a design process that could prove helpful even if carried out entirely on paper without using the computer at all.

Acknowledgments. Dr. Miller is supported in part by NIH grant R01 LM04336 from the National Library of Medicine. Dr. Mars is supported by a Constantijn en Christiaan Huygens Fellowship from the Dutch Organization for the Advancement of Pure Research (grant CCH 62-231).

References

1. Miller PL: A Critiquing Approach to Expert Computer Advice: ATTENDING. Boston: Pitman, 1984.
2. Miller PL: Expert Critiquing Systems: Practice-Based Medical Consultation by Computer. New York: Springer Verlag, 1986.
3. Miller PL, Black HR: Medical plan-analysis by computer: critiquing the pharmacologic management of essential hypertension. Comput Biomed Res 17:38, 1984.
4. Miller PL: Goal-directed critiquing by computer: ventilator management. Comput Biomed Res 18:422, 1985.
5. Miller PL, Blumenfrucht SJ, Black HR: An expert system which critiques patient workup: modeling conflicting expertise. Comput Biomed Res 17:554, 1984.
6. Miller PL, Shaw C, Rose JR, Swett HA: Critiquing the process of radiologic differential diagnosis. Comput Methods Programs Biomed 22:12, 1986.
7. Miller PL: Building an expert critiquing system: ESSENTIAL-ATTENDING. Methods Inf Med 25:71, 1986.
8. Davis R: Interactive transfer of expertise. p. 171. In Buchanan BG, Shortliffe EH (eds): Rule-Based Expert Systems. Reading, MA: Addison-Wesley, 1984.
9. Musen MA, Fagan LM, Combs DM, Shortliffe EH: Facilitating knowledge entry for an oncology therapy advisor using a model of the application area. In: Proceedings of MEDINFO-86, Washington, DC, 1986.
10. Politakis PG: Empirical Analysis for Expert Systems. Boston: Pitman, 1985.
11. Mars NJI, Miller PL: Knowledge acquisition and verification tools for medical expert systems. Med Decis Making 7:6, 1987.

15
Evaluation of Artificial Intelligence Systems in Medicine

Perry L. Miller

A number of projects have explored the application of artificial intelligence in medicine (AIM).[1-4] Many of these projects have resulted in the implementation of research prototype systems that explore fundamental computer science design issues. Recently a small number of systems have been introduced into clinical use.

The evaluation of AIM systems has always been an important part of their implementation. The appropriate form of evaluation, however, depends on a project's maturity and goals.[5] Evaluation of an AIM system might be performed at three levels.

1. Subjective assessment of the research contribution of a developmental system
2. Validation of a system's knowledge prior to possible clinical use
3. Evaluation of the clinical efficacy of an operational consultation system

This chapter examines the underlying issues confronted in these three forms of evaluation and discusses how several previous AIM evaluations fit into this framework.

Evaluating a Research Prototype System

For a research prototype system, appropriate evaluation may primarily involve the subjective assessment of the project's contribution to the field. This assessment includes such issues as the following.

New problems: Does the system uncover important new design problems that must be confronted in building an AIM system?
New solutions: Does the system offer design solutions to help deal with such problems?
New tools: Does the project develop tools to help researchers handle similar problems in other domains?

Illustrative mistakes: Does the system make illustrative mistakes that define interesting problems more fully and that help guide later work in constructive directions?

If the complexity of medical decision-making is approached in a scientific fashion, there must be projects that explore fundamental aspects of the various problems involved. Indeed, there may be a series of such systems as methodologies evolve, problems become more fully defined, promising domains are identified, and sufficiently powerful tools emerge.

The subjective evaluation of a developmental system is made by the system designers and by the field as a whole. Objective evaluation of early research prototypes may or may not be useful. Once the overall system design is complete, it may already be clear that the approach taken, or perhaps the domain itself, has significant practical limitations.

Clinical Validation of a System's Knowledge and Advice

The previous section discussed how a developmental AIM system may be evaluated subjectively, assessing its research contribution to the field. This section discusses how a developmental system might be "validated" based on more objective criteria. The issues dealt with in such a validation include the following.

Accuracy: Does the system include the knowledge its designers think it includes, i.e., is its knowledge "debugged"?

Completeness and consistency: Is the knowledge complete and consistent? Are there gaps or inconsistencies the system designers overlooked in their initial implementation?

Performance: If the system models a particular domain expert's knowledge, does it appropriately mirror that expert's performance?

Conflicting expertise: In many areas of medicine there are conflicting expert opinions as to appropriate practice, particularly in areas of medical management and work-up. When validating a system, one must decide how it should deal with conflicting expertise. Is the system to model one expert approach? Is it to incorporate more than one expert approach? If so, how?

What is the "gold standard"? Implicit in the issues of performance and conflicting expertise is the question of defining a "gold standard" against which to measure the system's performance. Medical decisions may involve a great deal of subjective judgment. Also, there may be great practice variation. As a result, it may be unclear whose individual or collective practice best serves as an appropriate standard of comparison. To validate a system, however, it must be determined. Some measure of interexpert agreement may help when developing realistic performance expectations.

Multiple categories of correctness: Just as there is difficulty defining a gold standard against which to compare a system's performance, there is potential ambiguity in interpreting when a diagnostic system has "correctly" produced a given diagnosis. Must the diagnosis be at the top of the system's differential? What if a patient has multiple diseases?

Limits of a system's expertise: Every expert system's knowledge is bounded. If a diagnostic system is presented with the manifestations of an unfamiliar disease, it should ideally fail to make a diagnosis and gracefully defer to another expert. If a system is tested using only familiar diseases, of course, this problem is never confronted.

Eliminating bias: When assessing a system's advice, there is clearly a potential for bias. Some evaluators may be skeptical of computer advice and may judge the system harshly. Others may be enthusiastic and forgiving of weaknesses. If possible, a validation must be designed to remove the potential for evaluator bias.

Efficient use of expert evaluators: The best evaluators of a system's advice are likely to be national and international experts in the field. Any system validation must therefore be designed to use their time efficiently.

Analyzing the causes of failure: If one compares a system's performance to some appropriate standard, one can gather statistics that measure how well it performs. Further insight may be gained, however, by analyzing in detail the reasons for any failures.

Knowledge Validation: Previous Experience

This section discusses several AIM evaluations that illustrate many of the issues outlined above.

MYCIN. MYCIN was developed at Stanford to determine diagnoses and recommend treatment for infectious diseases. Several evaluations of the system were performed. The most sophisticated tested a version of MYCIN in the domain of meningitis.[6]

Ten cases were selected based on a fairly complex set of criteria. For instance, the cases were to include, at most, three viral cases, and at least one tubercular, one fungal, one viral, and one bacterial case. These criteria helped ensure a representative sample of interesting cases while limiting the total number of cases (and the time demand placed on the expert evaluators).

For each of the ten cases, several treatment recommendations were obtained using (1) MYCIN, (2) Stanford infectious disease faculty, (3) an infectious disease fellow, (4) a resident, (4) a medical student, and (5) the actual therapy used for treating the patient. These different recommendations were then arranged in random order before being presented to outside expert evaluators, thereby helping remove any potential for bias.

The eight evaluators individually indicated how they would have treated each patient. They then ranked each proposed recommendation as either: (1) identical or equivalent to their own; (2) acceptable; or (3) unacceptable. Most of the evaluators approved MYCIN's choice 70 percent of the time. None of the other prescribers (including the Stanford infectious disease faculty) achieved better approval than MYCIN. Thus by including these other treatment recommendations s as a standard of comparison, it could be demonstrated that MYCIN's 70 percent approval was respectable.

AI/RHEUM. The AI/RHEUM system,[7] which determines rheumatologic diagnoses, was developed at the University of Missouri using the EXPERT system[8] of Rutgers. An initial retrospective study with 384 cases demonstrated an accuracy of 94 percent using the treating clinicians' diagnosis as a standard of comparison. In part to test the accuracy of this "gold standard," the raw data from 48 cases were subsequently presented to three rheumatologists. All three agreed on 28 cases. A majority agreed on 46 cases. This second study also served to confirm that the data being input to AI/RHEUM was sufficient to allow reliable diagnosis.

A third, prospective study was performed with 74 patients. Of them, 63 had diseases known to the system. All 63 were correctly diagnosed. The diseases of the remaining 11 patients were not known to the system. Of the 11, 7 were diagnosed incorrectly, and 4 were not diagnosed. This study highlights the problems that can occur at the limits of a system's knowledge when randomly selected cases include diseases unfamiliar to the system.

An additional issue addressed in these studies is that of "multiple categories of correctness" (and "incorrectness"). For instance, it is clear that not obtaining a diagnosis is different from diagnosing a patient incorrectly. Also, it is not always obvious how a "correct diagnosis" is best defined, especially in a patient with multiple diseases. In these studies a single diagnosis was considered correct if it was at the top (or tied at the top) of the system's differential. A patient with multiple diseases, however, was considered correctly diagnosed if all diseases were listed somewhere in the system's differential.

INTERNIST. The evaluation of the INTERNIST system,[9] whose domain is internal medicine, used clinicopathologic conferences from the *New England Journal of Medicine*. The standard of comparison was the performance of clinicians and discussants as documented in the journal. INTERNIST demonstrated impressive performance on these difficult cases. Of the 43 possible major diagnoses, INTERNIST made 17 definitively, the clinicians made 23, and the discussants made 29.

An interesting feature of this study was the explicit attention focused on the *reasons* for the system's failures. Some of these failures had a clearly different character from the problems human diagnosticians have. These failures arose from limitations in the system's knowledge and in its diagnostic algorithms, and led to a detailed discussion of how the system might be refined, e.g., by addition of temporal, causal, anatomic, and physiologic knowledge.

SPE. SPE was developed at Rutgers to interpret the results of serum protein electrophoresis data produced by a laboratory instrument.[10] Although its published description is not detailed, this evaluation involved 256 cases. The standard of comparison was the expert who helped develop the system and an outside expert. The study is almost unique in AIM evaluations to date in that the system was judged to be 100 percent acceptable, with the disclaimer: "They [the experts] expect differences of opinion on the amount of detail included in the present set of conclusions, but feel that covering infrequently found problems in a more detailed manner would detract from a model that is to be disseminated widely." This study therefore suggests that in a sufficiently constrained domain, with clinically reasonable constraints on the scope of a system's advice, one may avoid certain "gold standard" problems of practice variation and conflicting expertise that figure so prominently in many evaluations.

TIA System. The TIA system was developed at the University of Maryland to help assess transient ichemic attacks (TIAs) and to recommend therapy.[11] The system's goal was to reproduce the decision-making of stroke specialists at that institution. In a retrospective study of 103 patients, the system's localization and classification performance was compared to that of the stroke specialists who saw each patient. In this part of the study, the system performed well. Interestingly, when the 12 cases where localization disagreement occurred were reviewed, the expert reviewer agreed with the system in 11 of the 12 cases.

In the same study, the TIA system's management recommendations were compared to those of the patients' physicians (whose treatment was not directly controlled by stroke specialists). Here there was considerable disagreement. These differences were difficult to assess for several reasons: (1) The treating physicians were not neurologists. (2) There is considerable difference of opinion as to management even among neurologists. (3) Some patients had been treated prior to publication of controlled trials of aspirin therapy, and others had been treated afterward. The system designers interpreted this disagreement, in part, as demonstrating the potential value of an expert TIA consultation system for nonstroke specialists.

Automating the Process of Knowledge Validation

An interesting approach to knowledge validation involves designing the system itself to assist in the process. Knowledge validation tools can operate in two general ways. (1) The system can inspect its own knowledge, searching for areas of inconsistency or incompleteness. (2) The system can facilitate such inspection by the system implementers. Such knowledge validation tools will form an important part of sophisticated AIM systems of the future.

One example of a knowledge validation tool is the rule checking program of ONCOCIN.[12] Another example is SEEK.[13] SEEK operates on the knowledge of a rule-based diagnostic system. It uses a set of stored cases, whose diagnoses are known, to guide its inspection of the system's knowledge. From this inspection, SEEK can hypothesize modifications of the rules (the diagnostic knowledge base) that might improve the system's diagnostic performance. The system designers can then decide if the suggested modifications make clinical sense.

Tutorial Use as a Modality for Knowledge Validation

Another approach to help validate a system's knowledge is to adapt the system for teaching while it is still under development for eventual consultation use. For instance, the prototype ATTENDING system,[14] which critiques anesthetic management, was adapted experimentally for teaching.[15] In its teaching mode the system presents hypothetical cases to a user who then proposes an anesthetic management plan for the system to critique.

Tutorial use can help exercise a system's knowledge and thereby flush out areas of weakness. Because a consultation system is not developed primarily for teaching, however, the system may not prove optimally designed for use as a teaching tool.

Evaluation of an Operational System's Clinical Efficacy

A further stage in evaluation involves objective and subjective measures of an operational system's clinical efficacy. Such an evaluation might be performed at several stages of system implementation, including: (1) experimental system use in a "protected" environment; (2) routine system use at a limited number of sites; or (3) widely disseminated system use. The specific issues addressed depend on the nature of the system, the domain, and the clinical role the system is asked to play. These issues include the following.

Physician actions: Does the physician-user alter his or her behavior based on the system's advice? For example, do diagnoses or treatment decisions change when the system is used?

Patient care: Is patient care improved based on objective standards such as fewer misdiagnoses or fewer management errors?

Patient health: The most fundamental issue, and sometimes the most difficult to measure, concerns the impact of a system on patient health.

For instance, if the system advises on antihypertensive treatment, are blood pressures better controlled or adverse side effects lessened when the system is used?

Health care process: Aside from its effect on patient care, a system may affect the overall health care delivery process: fewer lost records, better record-keeping, more efficient use of provider time, etc.

Cost/benefit analysis: Another important measure is the system's economic cost-effectiveness.

Subjective reactions: In addition to objective measures of effectiveness, one can elicit subjective reactions from people involved with the system: physicians, ancillary personnel, patients, etc.

User interface: One important feature central to a system's acceptance is the software– and hardware–user interface.

System use: The ultimate test of many systems, especially those whose use is optional, is if physicians find them useful and continue to use them.

Peer review: Another possibility is the formal evaluation of a system by expert reviewers. Because a consultation system represents a form of publication, it is reasonable that such systems undergo review similar to that performed for other types of publication.

Limitations of current technology: Another issue concerns the limitations of current technology. A system might be slow or awkward with existing hardware but acceptable using more advanced technology. If so, one would like to separate the evaluation of the system design, from any limitations imposed solely by current technology.

Clinical Evaluation of an Operational System: Previous Experience

The clinical evaluation of operational AIM systems remains largely unexplored, as few are currently in routine use.

ONCOCIN. The only AIM system known to the author to have undergone such an evaluation is ONCOCIN. ONCOCIN is designed to assist in oncology protocols and has been in routine experimental use at Stanford's oncology clinic. Two evaluations of this system's performance have been performed.

One study[16] is a knowledge validation of the working system. Here ONCOCIN's recommendations were compared to the treatment actually given. Any discrepancies were referred to expert analysis. Although both the system's advice and the treatments actually given were judged to be equally acceptable in most cases, certain specific areas of divergence were identified, especially in the degree of dosage attenuation and the length of treatment delays. These findings reflect the fact that even detailed oncology protocols (which form the basis for ONCOCIN's analysis) do not fully capture clinician expertise.

A second study[17] analyzed ONCOCIN's impact on a particular aspect of the health care delivery process: the frequency with which relevant clinical data were recorded. This study compared patient encounters before and after the introduction of ONCOCIN, including post-ONCOCIN encounters when the system was not available. The study demonstrated significantly increased recording of relevant data when the system was used. When the system was not available, recording tended to fall back to previous levels.

Assessing Clinical Efficacy in Developmental Systems. Certain of the issues outlined at the beginning of this section can be explored in a limited fashion in systems that are still developmental. One cannot, of course, draw as strong conclusions from such a system as one might from a fully operational system.

An example is the Digitalis Advisor[18] developed to assist with digitalis therapy. A 1-month preliminary evaluation of that system was performed using cardiology inpatients. In this study the system was not used to guide treatment but was tested in parallel to the patients' ongoing treatment. An interesting finding was that the system was able to detect digitalis toxicity earlier than the treating physicians.

Initial Choice of a Domain: A Central Evaluation Issue

Evaluation is often perceived as occurring late in a system's implementation. The most important determinant of an evaluation's success, however, may be the *initial choice* of an appropriate domain and of an appropriate role for the system to play in that domain.

To facilitate successful evaluation, a system's domain must be sufficiently constrained. The three AIM systems currently in routine clinical use, for instance, operate in domains that are significantly constrained. PUFF,[19] which interprets pulmonary function tests, and SPE,[10] which interprets serum electrophoresis data, are both constrained in that they interpret the output of laboratory instruments. (Because of this limitation, PUFF and SPE are not true *consultation* systems, as the physician does not use them interactively.) ONCOCIN,[20] which assists with oncology protocols, operates in a domain where existing chemotherapy protocols outline in detail how treatment is to proceed. As a result, ONCOCIN's knowledge acquisition is greatly facilitated, as is user acceptance of its advice.

Identifying a constrained domain and defining an appropriate role for the system to play are therefore central issues in the eventual success of a system evaluation.

Summary: Evaluation of AIM Systems, an Open Research Area

This chapter outlined a number of issues involved in the evaluation of AIM systems. System evaluation is clearly not a simple process.[5] A number of complex problems must be confronted. The evaluation may take different forms depending on such issues as the:

1. Maturity of the system design
2. Character of the domain
3. Type of advice the system gives
4. Clinical role the system is asked to play
5. Degree of agreement or disagreement among domain experts themselves
6. Goals of the project

Appropriate evaluation must therefore be tailored to a particular system. The field has only scratched the surface of many of the issues involved. New issues are bound to arise as increasingly complex AIM system are brought to the level of validation and clinical evaluation. As a result, the evaluation of AIM systems is an open research area and will remain so for the forseeable future.

Acknowledgment. This research was supported in part of NIH grant 03978 from the National Library of Medicine.

References

1. Shortliffe EH, Buchanan BG, Feigenbaum EA: Knowledge engineering for medical decision making: a review of computer-based clinical decision aids. Proc IEEE 67:1207, 1979.
2. Kulikowski C: Artificial intelligence methods and systems for medical consultation. IEEE Trans PAMI PAMI-2:464, 1980.
3. Szolovits P (ed): Artificial Intelligence in Medicine. Boulder, CO: Westview Press, 1982.
4. Clancey WJ, Shortliffe EH (eds): Readings in Medical Artificial Intelligence: The First Decade. Reading, MA: Addison-Wesley, 1984.
5. Buchanan BG, Shortliffe EH (eds): Rule-Based Expert Systems. Reading, MA: Addison-Wesley, 1984, p. 571.
6. Yu VL, Fagan LM, Wraith SM, Clancey WJ, Scott AC, Hannigan J, Blum RL, Buchanan BG, Cohen SN: Antimicrobial selection by a computer: a blinded evaluation by infectious disease experts. JAMA 242:1279, 1979.
7. Kingsland L, Sharp G, Capps R, Benge J, Kay D, Reese G, Hazelwood S, Lindberg D: Testing a criteria-based consultant system in rheumatology. p. 514. In: Proceedings of MEDINFO-83, Amsterdam, 1983.
8. Weiss SM, Kulikowski CA: EXPERT: a system for developing consultation models. p. 942. In: Proceedings of the Sixth International Joint Conference on Artificial Intelligence. Tokyo, 1979.

9. Miller RA, Pople HE, Myers JD: INTERNIST-1, an experimental computer-based diagnostic consultant for general internal medicine. N Engl J Med 307:468, 1982.
10. Weiss SM, Kulikowski CA, Galen RS: Representing expertise in a computer program: the serum protein diagnostic program. J Clin Lab Automation 3:383, 1983.
11. Reggia JA, Tabb DR, Price TR, Banko M, Hebel R: Computer-aided assessment of transient ischemic attacks: a clinical evaluation. Arch Neurol 41:1248, 1984.
12. Suwa M, Scott AC, Shortliffe EH: Completeness and consistency in a rule-based system. p. 159. In Buchanan BG, Shortliffe EH (eds): Rule-Based Expert Systems. Reading, MA: Addison-Wesley, 1984.
13. Politakis P, Weiss SM: A system for empirical experimentation with expert knowledge. p. 426. In Clancey WJ, Shortliffe EH (eds): Readings in Medical Artificial Intelligence: The First Decade. Addison-Wesley, Reading, MA: 1984.
14. Miller PL: A Critiquing Approach to Expert Computer Advice: ATTENDING. Boston: Pitman, 1984.
15. Miller PL, Angers D, Keefer JR, Sudan N, Tanner G: Teaching with "ATTENDING": tutorial use of an expert system. p. 87. In: Proceedings of AAMSI CONGRESS-83, San Francisco, 1983.
16. Hickam DH, Shortliffe EH, Bischoff MB, Scott AC, Jacobs CD: A study of the treatment advice of a computer-based cancer chemotherapy protocol advisor. Ann Intern Med 103:928, 1985.
17. Kent DL, Shortliffe EH, Carlson RW, Bischoff MB, Jacobs CD: Improvements in data collection through physician use of a computer-based chemotherapy treatment consultant. J Clin Oncol 3:1409, 1985.
18. Gorry GA, Silverman H, Pauker SG: Capturing clinical expertise: a computer program that considers clinical responses to digitalis. Am J Med 64:452, 1978.
19. Aikins JS, Kunz JC, Shortliffe EH, Fallat RJ: PUFF: an expert system for interpretation of pulmonary function data. Comput Biomed Res 16:199, 1983.
20. Shortliffe EH, Scott AC, Bischoff MB, Campbell AB, van Melle W, Jacobs CD: An expert system for oncology protocol management. p. 653. In Buchanan BG, Shortliffe EH (eds): Rule-Based Expert Systems. Reading, MA: Addison-Wesley, 1984.

16
Evaluation of Medical Expert Systems: Experience with the AI/RHEUM Knowledge-Based Consultant System in Rheumatology

Lawrence C. Kingsland III

The AI/RHEUM diagnostic consultant system was developed as a multidisciplinary project involving the Information Science Group and the Division of Immunology/Rheumatology at the University of Missouri School of Medicine in Columbia and the Department of Computer Science at Rutgers University.[1-3] The project objective for AI/RHEUM has been to produce a computer-based rheumatology consultant having performance at the level of an expert rheumatologist. Its intended users are practicing physicians not having specialty training in rheumatology, though the system's use in the education of medical students and house staff is envisioned.

The AI/RHEUM knowledge base derives from formal criteria[4-6] for 26 rheumatologic diseases. The system reasons from a patient data checklist of 877 elements, through 652 intermediate hypotheses and 1029 production rules, to its 26 disease conclusions. It has been tested with more than 500 carefully studied clinical cases.

Methods

AI/RHEUM runs under the EXPERT system[7] developed by Kulikowski, Weiss, and Kern at Rutgers University. EXPERT uses production rules in a causal-inferential network, allowing AI/RHEUM to reason from patient findings through intermediate hypotheses to disease hypotheses. The patient findings consist of basic information such as signs, symptoms, laboratory test results, and radiographic observations. Intermediate hypotheses are combinations of findings, usually representing pathophysiologic states (e.g., serious central nervous system involvement) or useful aggregates of observations. An intermediate hypothesis may be combined with additional findings or with other intermediate hypotheses to generate further intermediate hypotheses, to an arbitrary number of levels. Disease hypotheses are the final step in the model's reasoning.

For patient findings that may be unfamiliar to physicians trained in nonrheumatologic specialties, AI/RHEUM has available on line a series of text definitions invoked by a "Tell me more" command. Many of the definitions offer four categories of explanation: WHAT (is this observation), WHY (is the observation being requested), HOW (is the observation performed), and REFS (citations from the medical literature). There are 172 definitions on line in the current model. The intent of this facility is to improve the likelihood that accurate observations will be input to AI/RHEUM and to enhance the educational potential of the system.

When the text explanation of a finding unfamiliar to the user is not sufficient, the user of AI/RHEUM can trigger the "Show me more" command to display images from an interactive videodisc system directly linked to the consultant system. The videodisc contains 1900 still-frame images representing examples of many of the findings requested by AI/RHEUM.

For current information in the form of citations from the world's biomedical literature, the user can invoke the "Search for more" option in AI/RHEUM. This command loads the National Library of Medicine's personal computer (PC)-based front end system, GRATEFUL MED, for searching the 6.5 million records of the MEDLINE files. GRATEFUL MED performs an auto-dialout and auto-logon, assists the user with the formulation of the query, performs the MEDLINE search, downloads the results (with abstracts, if requested), logs off, and returns control to AI/RHEUM.

For each disease in the system's knowledge base, formal criteria are defined. The criteria contain major and minor decision elements, required decision elements ("must have" items), and exclusions ("must not have" items). Each of these decision elements in the criteria may be an individual patient finding or an intermediate hypothesis, potentially a complex combination of many findings. The disease criteria are the consensus of discussions among clinicians from the Division of Immunology/Rheumatology at the University of Missouri–Columbia School of Medicine after study of the published literature, with periodic review by an external panel of nationally known rheumatologists. The 26 diseases for which criteria have been defined in the AI/RHEUM knowledge base have been listed in other reports.[1-3] The criteria tables themselves are also available on line to the system user. They constitute the fourth knowledge source ("Tell me more" text definitions, "Show me more" video images, "Search for more" MEDLINE citations, disease criteria tables) directly accessible from the running program.

As the number of diseases in the knowledge base grew, it seemed increasingly important to give the user a medically sound output statement that would engender some confidence that the system's reasoning was based on identifiable clinical knowledge. The current AI/RHEUM output is a set of disease hypotheses in a differential diagnosis. Each component of the differential is further characterized as definite, probable, or possible. A summary of the reasoning that generated each component in the differential diagnosis is presented in terms of (1) findings that support the diagnosis; (2) findings positive for the patient that are *not* explained by this diagnosis; and (3) findings presently unknown, which if known and positive would tend to strengthen the diagnosis.

The list of findings currently unknown is presented ranked along a spectrum from findings inexpensive, easy, and safe for the patient (e.g., body temperature) to findings expensive, difficult, and potentially hazardous (e.g., renal biopsy). This ordered list constitutes a graded series of suggested next tests, the results of which would allow the system better to focus its differential diagnosis. An example of the AI/RHEUM output for one of the cases tested is presented in Table 16.1.

Several key parameters of the growing model over the years of its development are presented in Table 16.2, which shows the increase in various components of the system (number of diseases, findings, intermediate hy-

Table 16.1. Example of AI/RHEUM Output

Diagnoses are considered in the categories *definite, probable,* and *possible.*
Based on the information provided, the differential diagnosis is
    Sjögren's syndrome—*definite*
    Rheumatoid arthritis—*possible*
Diagnosis of Sjögren's syndrome is supported by the patient findings
    Keratoconjunctivitis sicca
    Xerostomia
    RA factor positive
Unknown findings that would help support the diagnosis of Sjögren's syndrome
    Parotid enlargement
    FANA positive
    Lip bx for Sjögren's positive
Diagnosis of rheumatoid arthritis is supported by the patient findings
    Chronic symmetric polyarthritis >6 weeks
    Joint deformity
    ESR Westergren >30 mm/hr
    RA factor positive
    Morning stiffness
Findings not explained by the diagnosis rheumatoid arthritis
    Diarrheal illness within last 2 weeks
Unknown findings that would help support the diagnosis of rheumatoid arthritis
    Subcutaneous rheumatoid nodules
    Synovial fluid, inflammatory
    Synovial biopsy, rheumatoid changes

---

bx, biopsy; FANA, fluorescent antinuclear antibody; RA, rheumatoid arthritis.

Table 16.2. Growth of the AI/RHEUM Model

Model	Dis	Find	IHyp	Rules	Pages
RH0380	7	151	38	123	8+
RH0181	11	679	90	310	27+
RH0281	14	679	109	360	29+
RH0381	16	679	124	400	32+
RH0481	20	763	374	774	38+
RH0282	26	875	464	1014	55+
RH0283	26	877	467	1017	167+
RH0186	26	877	652	1029	194+

See text for explanation of abbreviations.

potheses, rules, and pages of source statements in the uncompiled model) as the knowledge base became more comprehensive. The model called RH0380 was the final connective tissue disease version before expansion of the knowledge base to other areas of rheumatology. This model's diagnosis agreed with a consensus of rheumatologists in 142 of 156 training cases (91 percent), and in 99 of 104 independent testing cases (95 percent). The model called RH0186 is the current 26-disease version. An experimental 32-disease version now being tested will be reported in subsequent manuscripts.

Results

The AI/RHEUM diagnostic model has from its inception been challenged with actual clinical cases. Initially, the cases were taken from retrospective chart reviews selected specifically because the patients carried discharge diagnoses that occurred in the model's knowledge base. The results of this testing for 384 carefully studied clinical cases are found in Table 16.3.

Table 16.3. Diagnostic Accuracy of AI/RHEUM, Selected Cases

Diagnosis	Cases Correct	
Connective tissue diseases	235/254	(93%)
Spondyloarthropathies	34/34	(100%)
Crystal-induced arthritides	19/19	(100%)
Infection-induced arthritides	29/30	(97%)
Juvenile rheumatoid arthritis	17/17	(100%)
Other rheumatalogic disorders	26/30	(87%)
Overall, all cases	360/384	(94%)

When judging the accuracy of the AI/RHEUM model, we compared
the differential diagnosis in its output statement with the presumptive "gold
standard" diagnosis of a consensus of expert rheumatologist-clinicians.
To test the repeatability of this "gold standard," we conducted a blinded
review of a group of sample cases from the AI/RHEUM data base. We
printed unidentified raw case summaries from the patient data base and
had them reviewed independently by three rheumatologists. Of 48 such
summaries reviewed, all three clinicians agreed on the diagnosis for 28
cases, and two of three agreed on the diagnosis for an additional 18 cases.
Thus at least two of three rheumatologists agreed on the diagnosis of 46
of the 48 cases, an impressive consistency of 96 percent for these difficult
clinical cases. The standard did seem valid.

AI/RHEUM had been tested during its development with 384 selected
cases. We now determined to test the system with unselected cases in
order to derive some experience with the coverage afforded in a real-
world rheumatology ward situation by the 26 diseases in the knowledge
base. The system was challenged with all but one (one chart had been
lost) of the cases admitted to the Arthritis Unit at the University of Missouri–Columbia over two specific 60-day periods. For 74 cases admitted
during October and November of 1981 and 1982, we filled out patient data
checklists, entered the information into the model, and recorded the differential diagnosis produced by AI/RHEUM. The results of this unselected
test series are presented in Table 16.4.

The results were better than we had hoped. Of this unselected group
of 74 cases, 63 carried diagnoses represented in the AI/RHEUM knowledge
base (85 percent). All 63 cases having diagnoses known to the system
were in fact correctly diagnosed by the system. Of the 11 cases that had
diagnoses not represented in the knowledge base (KB), AI/RHEUM appropriately refused to make any diagnostic conclusion on five. The system
was misled by features of diseases it knew on the other cases, misdi-
agnosing the final six. Of the five cases for which AI/RHEUM had refused
to state a differential diagnosis for lack of sufficient evidence, two had

Table 16.4. Diagnostic Accuracy of AI/
RHEUM, Unselected Cases

Model Diagnosis	Clinical Diagnosis in KB	Clinical Diagnosis Not in KB
Correct	63	NA
Incorrect	0	6
None given	0	5

for the same reason been left without specific diagnoses by the clinicians. In summary, 63 of 74 cases were diagnosed correctly by AI/RHEUM (85 percent); in 68 of 74 cases the model made an appropriate statement (92 percent); and 6 of 74 cases the model simply was wrong (8 percent).

The 11 diagnoses AI/RHEUM missed because they were lacking in the knowledge base are presented in Table 16.5. Some of these diagnoses, e.g., monoarticular arthritis of unknown etiology, are rather nebulous attempts by the attending physician to apply a diagnostic label to a vague, undifferentiated case in which there obviously was little to go on. Though there was not enough evidence to make a real diagnosis, the physicians were able to specify something of what they did know. Our system's statement that the evidence was insufficient to warrant a diagnostic conclusion is more straightforward but less helpful. Perhaps we must work on an output statement of the form, "We cannot assign a diagnosis to this case, but we do know that the patient shows signs of problems X, Y, and Z."

We had now tested AI/RHEUM with 384 selected cases and 74 unselected cases, largely from the University of Missouri Hospital and Clinics. Further testing was necessary to determine if we had been able to avoid a parochial bias in the knowledge base: if cases sent to AI/RHEUM from a wholly different environment would be handled as successfully. We were fortunate that a group of rheumatologist clinicians from Keio University in Japan agreed to fill out patient data checklists and send us a series of test cases. This series ultimately consisted of 59 difficult connective tissue disease cases, many carrying multiple diagnoses. The results of this test series are shown in Table 16.6.

Table 16.5 Unselected Cases, Diagnosis Not Known to AI/RHEUM

Monoarticular arthritis, ? etiology
Hypothyroidism
Relapsing polychondritis
Reactive arthritis
Reflex sympathetic dystrophy
Anxiety neurosis
Eosinophilic fasciitis
Clubbing, ? etiology
Peripheral neuropathy, ? etiology
Behçet's disease
Essential mixed cryoglobulinemia

Table 16.6. Diagnostic Accuracy of AI/RHEUM,
Japanese Cases

Cases	No.	
Correct	54/59	(92%)
Partially correct three- and four-diagnosis cases; all but one diagnosis found in model's differential)	3/59	(5%)
Incorrect	2/59	(3%)

Discussion

A number of factors warrant thought and effort in the testing of clinical consulting systems such as AI/RHEUM.[8–10] Of primary importance is the existence of a known correct diagnosis against which the computer system's conclusions may be compared. The blinded case review reported above represents our effort to ensure that expert clinicians are in fact able to establish correct diagnoses solely on the basis of the information available to the model. It implies that the information present is also sufficient for the model to reach a corresponding diagnosis, provided the disease criteria tables in its knowledge base adequately represent the knowledge used by the clinicians in reaching the correct diagnosis. The analysis of errors made by the model determines if disease criteria should be amended. During the development of the criteria, one can learn more from cases initially misdiagnosed by the model than from those correctly handled on the first pass.

As useful as a "gold standard" diagnosis would be a set of benchmark cases containing classic examples of each disease in the knowledge base. In the records of a tertiary care referral center, many cases are atypical in their complexity. We have not yet sufficiently tested the hypothesis that a system that can handle difficult cases will have no trouble with the more prevalent simple ones.

Even with a "gold standard" in hand, the scoring of a consultant system may be more complex than expected. When comparing AI/RHEUM's diagnostic statement with that of the clinicians, we scored the model as correct when it presented the clinicians' diagnosis at the top level of its differential diagnosis or tied with other diagnoses at the top level. The model was scored incorrect when it did not present the clinicians' diagnosis in the top level of its differential, even in cases in which it included this correct diagnosis at a lower confidence level elsewhere in the differential diagnosis portion of its output statement. For cases carrying multiple rheumatologic diagnoses, the model in the retrospective testing was scored correct only when all of the clinicians' diagnoses that were in its knowledge base appeared in its differential statement. In the unselected testing, a case was scored wholly correct only when all of the rheumatologic diseases in its clinical diagnosis were both represented in the model's knowledge base and included in the model's differential diagnosis for that case.

Miller and co-workers noted when reporting on a trial of INTERNIST-1[11] that failure to make a correct diagnosis is not the same as making an incorrect diagnosis. There are in fact multiple categories of correctness in the scoring of systems such as these. A case may be carrying several diagnoses, not all of which are represented in the model's knowledge base. Scoring of the system's performance then must account for numerous combinations of the five potential outcomes shown in Table 16.7.

During our testing, we encountered several cases in which AI/RHEUM came to specific disease conclusions not carried on the patient's chart. On careful review, we found that the patient findings present justified the model's conclusion: The model was correct. In some such cases the clinician had made the primary diagnosis and missed a secondary diagnosis. There may be occasions on which a clinician, having assigned a diagnosis to a particular case, fails to pursue findings not explained by the primary diagnosis that would lead to the secondary conclusion. AI/RHEUM pursues all the possibilities, evaluating each finding in terms of all the sets of disease criteria in its knowledge base.

Though we have in this discussion concentrated on issues of diagnostic accuracy, other steps are equally important to a comprehensive system evaluation. Shortliffe and Clancey[12] suggested seven steps: (1) demonstrate a need for the system; (2) demonstrate that the system performs at the level of an expert; (3) demonstrate the system's usability; (4) demonstrate acceptance of the system by physicians; (5) demonstrate an impact on the management of patients; (6) demonstrate an impact on the well-being of patients; (7) demonstrate cost-effectiveness of the tool. The further statement by Shortliffe and Clancey that, "We know of no medical decision-making system that has rigorously been shown to meet formal validation criteria at all seven steps of development" is probably still true today.

Table 16.7. Potential Outcomes in Scoring

Dx in KB, correct conclusion by the model
Dx in KB, incorrect conclusion by the model
Dx in KB, incorrect refusal by the model to make a conclusion
Dx not in KB, correct refusal by the model to make a conclusion
Dx not in KB, incorrect conclusion by the model of a disease from its KB

Dx, diagnosis; KB, knowledge base.

The performance of the AI/RHEUM diagnostic consultant system to date (step 2—demonstrating that the system performs at the level of an expert) warrants its testing in additional clinical settings. The system has been ported from the DECsystem-20 at Rutgers to the VAX-11/780's in-house at the Lister Hill National Center for Biomedical Communications, the research and development division of the National Library of Medicine. With new versions of EXPERT and AI/RHEUM by the National Library of Medicine now running on the IBM PC AT under PC-DOS, significant enhancements to the user interface and specific links to four knowledge sources in varying forms have been added.[3] The further extension of the system and its formal evaluation as a test of a general methodology for the evaluation of medical expert systems are in process at the National Library of Medicine.

Acknowledgments. The AI/RHEUM system is the result of a profoundly rewarding collaboration among researchers from Dr. Donald A.B. Lindberg's Information Science Group and Dr. Gordon C. Sharp's Division of Immunology/Rheumatology at the University of Missouri in Columbia, and Dr. Casimir A. Kulikowski's Department of Computer Science at Rutgers, The State University of New Jersey. More than 30 persons have contributed significantly to the AI/RHEUM project over the course of its development. Their time, talents, and efforts have been instrumental in the production of this system.

This research was begun and the studies herein reported to be performed at the University of Missouri in Columbia were supported in part by grant DHHS 5T15 LM07006 from the National Library of Medicine and grant DHHS 5P60 AM20658 from the National Institute of Arthritis, Diabetes, and Digestive and Kidney Diseases. Dr. Lindberg and Dr. Kingsland are now at the National Library of Medicine, where the continued enhancement and evaluation of AI/RHEUM is taking place.

This chapter is an expansion of concepts presented initially elsewhere.[2]

References

1. Kingsland LC III, Roeseler GC, Lindberg DAB, Sharp GC, Kay DR, Weiss SM: An expert consultant system in rheumatology: AI/RHEUM. p. 748. In Blum BI (ed): Proceedings of the Sixth Annual Symposium on Computer Applications in Medical Care (SCAMC). New York: IEEE Computer Society, 1982.
2. Kingsland LC III, Sharp GC, Capps RC, Benge JM, Kay DR, Reese GR, Hazelwood SE, Lindberg DAB: Testing of a criteria-based consultant system in rheumatology. p. 514. In van Bemmel JH, Ball MJ, Wigertz O (eds): Proceedings of the Fourth World Conference on Medical Informatics (MEDINFO 83). Amsterdam: North Holland, 1983.
3. Kingsland LC III, Lindberg DAB, Sharp GC: Anatomy of a knowledge-based consultant system: AI/RHEUM. MD Comput 3(5):18, 1986.

4. Lindberg DAB, Kingsland LC III, Roeseler GC, Kay DR, Sharp GC: A new knowledge representation for diagnosis in rheumatology. p. 299. In Lindberg DAB, Collen MF, van Brunt EE (eds): Proceedings of the First AMIA Congress on Medical Informatics (AMIA Congress 82). New York: Masson, 1982.
5. Lindberg DAB, Kingsland LC III, Waugh W, Benge JM, Sharp GC: Criteria tables as a possible general knowledge representation. p. 187. In Lindberg DAB, Collen MF (eds): Proceedings of the Congress on Medical Informatics (AAMSI Congress 1984). Bethesda: American Association for Medical Systems and Informatics, 1984.
6. Kingsland LC III, Lindberg DAB: The criteria form of knowledge representation in medical artificial intelligence. p. 12. In Salamon R, Blum B, Jorgensen M (eds): Proceedings of the Fifth Conference on Medical Informatics (MEDINFO 86). Amsterdam: North Holland, 1986.
7. Weiss SM, Kulikowski CA: EXPERT: a system for developing consultation models. p. 942. In: Proceedings of the Sixth International Joint Conference on Artificial Intelligence (IJCAI-79). Los Altos, CA: William Kaufmann, 1979.
8. Flagle CD: Evaluation of health care. p. 46. In van Bemmel JH, Ball MJ, Wigertz O (eds): Proceedings of the Fourth World Conference on Medical Informatics (MEDINFO 83). Amsterdam: North Holland, 1983.
9. Gaschnig J, Klahr P, Pople H, Shortliffe E, Terry A: Evaluation of expert systems: issues and case studies. p. 241. In Hayes-Roth F, Waterman DA, Lenat DB (eds): Building Expert Systems. Reading, MA: Addison-Wesley, 1983.
10. Buchanan BG, Shortliffe EH: The problem of evaluation. p. 571. In Buchanan BG, Shortliffe EH (eds): Rule-Based Expert Systems: The MYCIN Experiments of the Stanford Heuristic Programming Project. Reading, MA: Addison-Wesley, 1984.
11. Miller RA, Pople HE, Myers JD: INTERNIST-1, an experimental computer-based diagnostic consultant for general internal medicine. N Engl J Med 307:468, 1982.
12. Shortliffe EH, Clancey WJ: Anticipating the second decade. p. 467. In Clancey WJ, Shortliffe EH (eds): Readings in Medical Artificial Intelligence: The First Decade. Reading, MA: Addison-Wesley, 1984.

17
Evaluation of Medical Expert Systems: Case Study in Performance Assessment
James A. Reggia

As with any new agent introduced into medical practice, a medical expert system must be critically evaluated for its safety and efficacy in a clinical setting prior to its use in patient care. Assessing expert system performance in this way is similar to data collection in that it can be a difficult and time-consuming process. At least three aspects of system performance can be considered*: accuracy, usefulness, and transferability.[2] In this section a framework for viewing expert system performance assessment is outlined. The next section illustrates the concepts involved by discussing the clinical evaluation of an expert system that assists with management of patients with transient ischemic attacks (TIAs). The final section identifies factors that were crucial in the efficient development and testing of the TIA expert system.

The first question to resolve about any medical expert system is its *accuracy*. Although it may initially be tested in an informal fashion or by using records from a series of appropriate previously seen patients, ideally a prospective, well constructed clinical evaluation is desirable. The nature of the predictions/classifications being made and whether the "correct" answer is known guide the selection of an appropriate approach to measuring accuracy.

Several methods have evolved for measuring the accuracy of medical expert system predictions when the correct decisions or answers are known. The traditional error rate approach involves simply counting the number of correct and incorrect classifications the system produces. For example, the *sensitivity* of a diagnostic expert system for a certain diagnosis can be defined as the number of times it correctly predicts that diagnosis to be present divided by the total number of times the disease occurs in the test population. Similarly, the *specificity* is the number of times the expert system correctly predicts a diagnosis to be absent divided by the

---

*An additional issue is the efficiency with which conclusions are reached.[1]

© 1985 by the Institute of Electrical and Electronics Engineers, Inc. Reprinted with permission from the *Proceedings of the 9th Annual Symposium on Computer Applications in Medical Care*, Washington, D.C., November, pp. 287–291.

total number of patients who are free of that disease in the test population. Other related concepts, including "ROC curves"[3] and "coincidence matrices,"[4] have been discussed extensively in the literature and used in practice.[5]

Traditional error rate techniques are appealing in their simplicity, but their application to measure expert system accuracy faces at least two limitations. First, for some clinical problems it is difficult to define a "correct" answer to compare with that made by a medical expert system. For example, this could occur if several expert physicians disagreed among themselves as to the most appropriate drug to use for a particular disease. In such a situation, it has been recommended that a clinical trial be undertaken where "blinded" experts comparatively score the performance of both the expert system and other physicians (i.e., without knowing which predictions or recommendations are from the expert system).[6] Alternatively, an expert system's conclusions can be compared informally to those of a panel of expert physicians.[7]

A more formal approach to situations where the correct answer is not always known is to statistically measure *agreement* between an expert system and some standard of correctness (e.g., an expert physician). The kappa statistic[8] and its weighted variant[9] provide a measurement of agreement (not accuracy) of this sort that subtracts out the percentage of agreements that could be accounted for by chance alone. In its simplest form kappa is given by

$$\kappa = \frac{P_o - P_c}{1 - P_c}$$

where P_o is the proportion of observed agreements between expert system and standard, and P_c is the proportion of agreements that could be attributed to chance. This statistic has the interpretation that $\kappa = 1.0$ indicates perfect agreement, $\kappa = 0$ indicates a level of agreement expected by chance alone, and $\kappa < 0$ indicates less than chance agreement.

The second limitation of traditional error rate techniques for measuring accuracy is that they do not take into account the probabilistic nature of many clinical problems. For example, if one expert system predicted that a patient had disease X with a probability of 0.75, and a second expert system also predicted that the patient had disease X but with a probability of 0.95, both systems would be counted as correct by traditional criteria if the patient did have disease X. Measuring accuracy in this fashion therefore loses information: it misses the fact that the second expert system was in some sense "more correct" than the first.

The use of "accuracy coefficients" that assess the magnitude of differences in predictions has been advocated as a solution to this problem.[10] For example, the accuracy coefficient

$$Q = (2/n) \sum_{i=1}^{n} (p_i - 0.5)$$

has been used in this fashion.[11] Here, n is the number of predictions being made (i.e., cases) and p_i is the probability assigned by the expert system to the outcome that actually occurred in the ith case. Q has the interpretation that a value of 1 equals perfect prediction, a value of 0 indicates no predictive skill, and a value of -1 indicates perfectly incorrect prediction. Note that error rate measurements may rank the accuracy of a set of expert systems in a different order than that of an accuracy coefficient, a phenomenon referred to as the "electoral college effect."[11]

If one is interested in any clinically meaningful use of a medical expert system, one must go beyond assessing its accuracy and also address *usefulness*. It must not only be shown that the system is accurate, but that it is more accurate than the intended users. At least one study has demonstrated that physicians can be influenced in a detrimental fashion by expert system predictions that are less accurate than their own predictions.[12] Furthermore, some indication that a medical expert system is cost-effective (e.g., decreases hospital stays) or has indirect benefits (e.g., educational, as with "critiquing systems"[13,14]) is needed if one anticipates convincing physicians of the system's value. Relatively little work has been done to prove that expert systems are useful when adopted in practice, although decreased medication toxicity,[15] decreased exploratory surgery,[16] and shortened hospital stays through prevention of drug interactions and adverse effects[17] provide some notable exceptions.

Finally, a third issue concerning medical expert system performance is the *transferability* of a system from its original development site to geographically distant sites. An expert system's transferability involves not only its physical portability but also its applicability in a new environment (e.g., adaptability to differences in generally accepted treatment approaches) and its accuracy. A few studies have demonstrated that at times medical expert systems can be transferred to a new, geographically distant institution and still provide accurate classifications[11,18] but much more work needs to be done in the area to clarify this possibility.

Evaluation of the TIA Expert System

A TIA is a temporary episode of focal neurologic deficit secondary to localized ischemia that lasts for less than 24 hours. Despite this simple definition, the clinical examination and treatment of patients who have TIAs are complex and controversial problems. In one study, 30% of the patients originally classified by their physician as having TIAs were reclassified as not having TIAs when their charts were subsequently reviewed by a stroke specialist.[19] In addition, surveys have revealed that younger neurologists perceive the management of TIAs and other cerebrovascular diseases to be a difficult problem,[20] and that physicians in general frequently are uncertain about how best to manage such patients.[21-23]

Because of the importance of TIAs and the frequency with which they are seen by physicians, as well as the difficulties noted above, we are exploring development of a computer-supported decision aid for the classification and management of TIAs. The long-term goal of this work is to provide an interactive computer system that is directly usable by a physician as an "intelligent textbook"[24] about TIAs. The immediate goal is much more modest: to demonstrate that rule-based deduction is able to capture and emulate the complex, judgmental decision criteria used by stroke specialists at our institution when localizing and classifying TIAs. In addition, we wanted to compare computer-generated recommendations for patient treatment with what was actually done for patients by nonstroke specialists to gain some perspective on the potential usefulness of such a decision aid.

The TIA expert system was built using KMS, a domain-independent expert system generator.[24] The consequent-driven rule-based component of KMS was utilized, itself modeled after the mixture of deductive and statistical techniques introduced in MYCIN.[25] Given a patient description, the TIA system makes a number of logical deductions about the patient and displays its conclusions to the physician. These conclusions include statements about the following criteria: (1) localization to the appropriate vascular distribution; (2) classification (definite, possible, or doubtful TIA); (3) results of screening for uncommon causes; (4) additional screening tests that would be appropriate; and (5) suggestions about patient treatment. The decision criteria used by the TIA system in each of these five areas are outlined in detail elsewhere.[26]

After the TIA expert system was functional, 103 patients previously referred to the University of Maryland Hospital (Baltimore) Stroke Service because of the suspicion of TIAs were selected to evaluate the TIA system. The purpose of this evaluation was to determine how accurately the TIA system reproduced the decision-making of stroke specialists at our institution. Seventy-eight of the 103 cases used to evaluate the TIA system were randomly selected from patients seen at our hospital during the years 1972 through 1975 as part of the TIA cooperative study.[27] Patients were originally identified for inclusion in the TIA cooperative study by exhaustive chart reviews: Any patient whose physician recorded a diagnosis of TIA was entered in the study, and his or her chart was reviewed by a stroke specialist (defined to be a neurologist on our stroke service). This neurologic review process resulted in 16 of these patients being classified by the stroke specialist as having definite TIAs, 23 being reclassified as having possible TIAs, and 39 being reclassified as having doubtful TIAs.

The remaining 25 patients used to evaluate the TIA system were all patients with TIAs who were seen at our institution during an 18-month period as part of the pilot study of a national stroke data bank during the years 1980 through 1981.[28] With the exception of one patient later classified as having a doubtful TIA, these patients had all been classified by neurologists as having definite TIAs based on the stroke data bank protocol.

Evaluation of how well the TIA system duplicated the localization and classification decisions of the stroke specialists at our institution who helped to create the program was measured by comparing its decisions with those recorded by the stroke specialist who had reviewed each of the 103 test cases. A weighted κ statistic (κ_w) was used to measure the extent of agreement between the TIA system and the stroke specialist involved for each of these decisions. As noted earlier, the κ_w statistic measures the agreement between two "judges" after accounting for chance agreement. The κ_w statistic also permits the incorporation of ratio-scaled degrees of disagreement ("disagreement weights") so that disagreements of various severities can be weighted accordingly.

Evaluation of how well the TIA system's patient-treatment recommendations duplicated those of the stroke specialists who helped to create it could not be fairly (objectively) assessed because the specialists usually had not had direct control over patient treatment and their opinions at the time regarding treatment were not recorded. Instead, we compared the TIA system's treatment recommendations with what was actually done for each patient by the nonstroke specialist physicians who were generally in charge of the patients' care (an internist or general neurologist). The κ_w statistic was again used to measure agreement. The purpose of this evaluation was to obtain a preliminary indication of whether the TIA system's recommendations (which reflect those of our stroke specialists) differed significantly from actual patient treatments by nonstroke specialists. Such a difference would be a prerequisite for the TIA system to eventually serve as a useful decision aid or educational tool in practice.

For other decisions made by the TIA system (suspected uncommon causes, mimicking disorders, or appropriate additional screening tests), our records did not explicitly record the stroke specialist's or other physician's opinion. Objective evaluation of this aspect of the TIA system's behavior was therefore omitted.

The results of this evaluation of the TIA system are presented in Tables 17.1 through 17.4. Table 17.1 shows localization results for the 62 patients where both stroke specialist and TIA system specified a localization. The number of agreements was statistically significant after correction for chance agreements ($\kappa_w = 0.79$; significant at $p < 0.0001$). Table 17.2 shows analogous classification results ($\kappa_w = 0.625$; significant at $p < 0.0001$). Although some (correctable) errors in the TIA system's knowledge base were detected, the system was generally observed to be accurate in reproducing the clinical deductive abilities of stroke specialists for localizing and classifying TIAs. Analysis of those cases where disagreements occurred revealed that the TIA system's deductions were, in general, appropriate. We believe these results are convincing because the TIA system

Table 17.1. Localization Results

Stroke Specialist	LC LC/VB	RC RC/VB	VB	CS	Total
LC LC/VB	18	0	1	2	21
RC RC/VB	0	20	4	0	24
VB	1	2	12	0	15
CS	0	1	1	0	2
Total	19	23	18	2	62

LC = left carotid distribution; RC = right carotid distribution; VB = vertebral basilar distribution; CS = either carotid distribution.

used fairly standard and generally accepted criteria for TIA classification and localization.

Because the stroke specialist reviewing each case usually did not have control over patient treatment, the TIA system's performance in recommending arteriography and treatment could only be contrasted objectively with what the patient's primary physician actually did. The results concerning arteriography are presented in Table 17.3 ($\kappa_w = 0.31$; significant at $p < 0.005$) and those concerning treatment are presented in Table 17.4 ($\kappa_w = 0.31$; $p < 0.005$). Although the patient-treatment decisions made by the TIA system and the patients' physicians were statistically correlated, there were many cases where the physician's actions differed from the treatment steps recommended by the TIA system. Our subjective analysis of these differences generally confirmed that the TIA system was performing the logical deductions that its authors intended it to perform. Thus the significant discrepancy between the TIA system's recommendations and the actions of physicians suggests at least the potential for an expert system of this sort to influence patient care by providing a "second opinion." Of course the TIA system as it currently exists reflects

Table 17.2. Classification Results

Stroke Specialist	TIA System Definite	Possible	Doubtful	Total
Definite	23	10	7	40
Possible	7	10	6	23
Doubtful	0	0	40	40
Total	30	20	53	103

Table 17.3. Decisions on Arteriography

	TIA System		
Actual	Recommended Consideration of Arteriogram	No Comment on Arteriogram	Total
Done	24	11	35
Not done	24	44	68
Total	48	55	103

generally accepted decision criteria only among stroke specialists at our institution, and not all neurologists would agree with these criteria. However, it would be relatively straigtforward to incorporate alternate decision-making criteria supplied by other physicians into the TIA systems so that it might provide a user with multiple opinions on the same patient. The important point this study demonstrates is that the artificial intelligence method used in the TIA system is powerful enough to represent such criteria in a form that can be processed by a machine.

Discussion

The first section of this chapter outlined a framework for viewing existing methods for measuring expert system performance. The evaluation of the TIA system illustrates many of the concepts involved. Because a "correct" localization and classification are often a matter of opinion, a weighted kappa statistic was applied to measure the agreement (not accuracy!) of the TIA system with stroke specialists who served as the authoritative standard. The same metric was used to assess the agreement between the TIA system and nonstroke specialists on patient management (arteriography and treatment). The results of the latter measurement of agreement on patient management suggests that the TIA system may be useful in clinical practice. The TIA system's knowledge base is currently undergoing

Table 17.4. Comparison of Treatment Decisions

	TIA System				
Actual	Nonspecific	Aspirin	AC	End	Total
Nonspecific	50	8	0	0	58
Aspirin	15	10	0	0	25
AC	2	4	1	0	7
End	4	4	1	3	12
Total	71	26	2	3	102

AC = anticongulant; End = endarterectomy.

revision, and we intend to subsequently evaluate its performance in a prospective trial.

Finally, it is significant that the development and testing of the TIA system took roughly a 6 man-month effort.[26] This finding is in marked contrast with estimates of the development time that would be necessary for such an effort. For example: "Even for the best understood problems, experienced researchers using the best understood techniques still require at least 5 man-years to develop a system that begins to be robust."[29] Our ability to rapidly construct and clinically evaluate the TIA system was largely due to two factors: An expert system generator was used to implement the TIA system,[24] and an existing "data base" of suitable patient records was readily available for system testing.[27,28] Thus a great deal of the work (implementation of inference mechanism and user interface, collection of data for test cases, etc). was already done before development of the TIA system even began. The increasing availability of expert system generator tools and data bases, including those available on microcomputers, suggests that a proliferation of medical expert systems can be anticipated during the next decade. Increased critical evaluation of those systems crucial if they are to help improve patient care.

Acknowledgment. Supported in part by NIH award NS16332.

References

1. Chandrasekaran B: On evaluating AI systems for medical diagnosis. In: Proceeding MEDCOMP '82. Philadelphia: IEEE, 1982.
2. Reggia J, Tuhrim S: An overview of computer-assisted medical decision making. In Reggia J, Tuhrim S (eds): Computer-Assisted Medical Decision Making. New York: Springer Verlag, 1985, pp. 3–45.
3. McNeil B, Keeler E, Adelstein S: Primer on certain elements of medical decision making. N Engl J Med 293:211, 1975.
4. Salamon R, Bernadet M, Samson M, Derouesne C, Gremy F: Bayesian method applied to decision making in neurology—methodological considerations. Methods Inf Med 15:174, 1976.
5. Miller R, Pople H, Myers J: INTERNIST-I, an experimental computer-based diagnostic consultant for general internal medicine. N Engl J Med 307: 468, 1982.
6. Yu VL, Fagan LM, Wraith SM, Clancey WJ, Scott AC, Hanningan J, Blum RL, Buchanan BG, Cohen SN: Antimicrobial selection by a computer—a blinded evaluation by infectious disease experts. JAMA 42:1279, 1979.
7. Weiss S, Kulikowski C, Safir A: Glaucoma consultation by computer. Comput Biol Med 8:25, 1978.
8. Spitzer R, Cohen J, Fleiss J, Endicott J: Quantification of agreement in psychiatric diagnosis. Arch Gen Psychiatry 17:83, 1967.
9. Cohen J: Weighted kappa. Psychol Bull 70:213, 1968.
10. Shapiro A: The evaluation of clinical predictions. N Engl J Med 296:1509, 1977.

11. Zagoria R, Reggia J: Transferability of medical decision support systems based on Bayesian classification. Med Decis Making 3:501, 1983.
12. Dannenberg A, Shapiro A, Fries J: Enhancement of clinical predictive ability by computer consultation. Methods Inf Med 18:10, 1979.
13. Miller P: Critiquing—a different approach to expert computer advice in medicine. p. 17. In: Proceedings Eighth Annual Symposium on Computer Application in Medical Care. Washington DC: IEEE, 1984.
14. Langlotz C, Shortliffe E: Adopting a consultation system to critique user plans. Int J Man-Machine Stud 19:479, 1983.
15. Jelliffe R, Buell J, Kalaba R: Reduction of digitalis toxicity by computer-assisted glycoside dosage regimens. Ann Intern Med 77:891, 1972.
16. DeDombal F: Computer-aided diagnosis of acute abdominal pain. Br Med J 2:9, 1972.
17. Pryor T, Gardner R, Clayton P, Warner H: The HELP system. p. 109. In Blum B (ed): Information Systems for Patient Care, New York: Springer Verlag, 1984.
18. Zoltie N, Horrocks J, deDombal F: Computer assisted diagnosis of dyspepsia—report of transferability of a system, with emphasis on early diagnosis of gastric cancer. Methods Inf Med 16:89, 1977.
19. Calanchini P, Swanson P, Gotshall R, Haerer A, Poshanzer D, Price T: Cooperative study of hospital frequency and character of transient ischemic attacks: IV. The reliability of diagnosis: JAMA 238:2029, 1977.
20. Fisher R, Hanley D, Whisnant J, Barnett H: Transient Ischemic Attacks. Read before the American Society for Neurological Investigation, San Francisco, 1981.
21. Haerer A, Gotshall R, Conneally P, Dyken M, Poshanzer D, Price T, Swanson P, Calanchini P: Cooperative study of hospital frequency and character of transient ischemic attacks. III. Variations in treatment. JAMA 238:142, 1977.
22. Swanson P, Calanchini P, Dyken M, Gotshall R, Haerer A, Poskanzer D, Price T, Conneally P: Cooperative study of hospital frequency and character of transient: ischemic attacks. II. Performance of angiography among six centers. JAMA 237:2202, 1977.
23. Toole, J, Howard G: Management of asymptomatic carotid artery murmur and transient ischemic attacks. Arch Neurol 38:443, 1981.
24. Reggia J, Pula T, Price T, and Perricone B: Towards an intelligent textbook of neurology. p. 190. In: Proceedings of the Fourth Annual Symposium on Computer Applications in Medical Care. New York: IEEE, 1980.
25. Shortliffe E: Computer-Based Medical Consultations: MYCIN New York: Elsevier, 1976.
26. Reggia J, Tabb R, Price T, Banko M, Hebel R: Computer-aided assessment of transient ischemic attacks. Arch Neurol 41:1248, 1984.
27. Dyken M, Conneally M, Haerer A, Gotshall R, Calanchini P, Poskanzer D, Price T, Swanson P: Cooperative study of hospital frequency and character of transient ischemic attacks. I. Background, organization, and clinical survey. JAMA 237:882, 1977.
28. Kunitz S, Havekost C, Gross C: Pilot data bank networks for neurological disorders, p. 793. In: Proceedings of the Third Annual Symposium on Computer Application in Medical Care. Long Beach, CA: IEEE, 1979.
29. Davis R: Expert systems: Where are we? Where do we go from here? Artif Intell Magazine, 3:3, 1982.

Index